Nursing scl
and wh

by

Stacey Bernikow

This book, my heart, and all my love is dedicated to my awesome kids, Leah, Jake and Rose.
You were my motivation and inspiration that got me thru three of the toughest years ever.
I love love love you!
-Mom

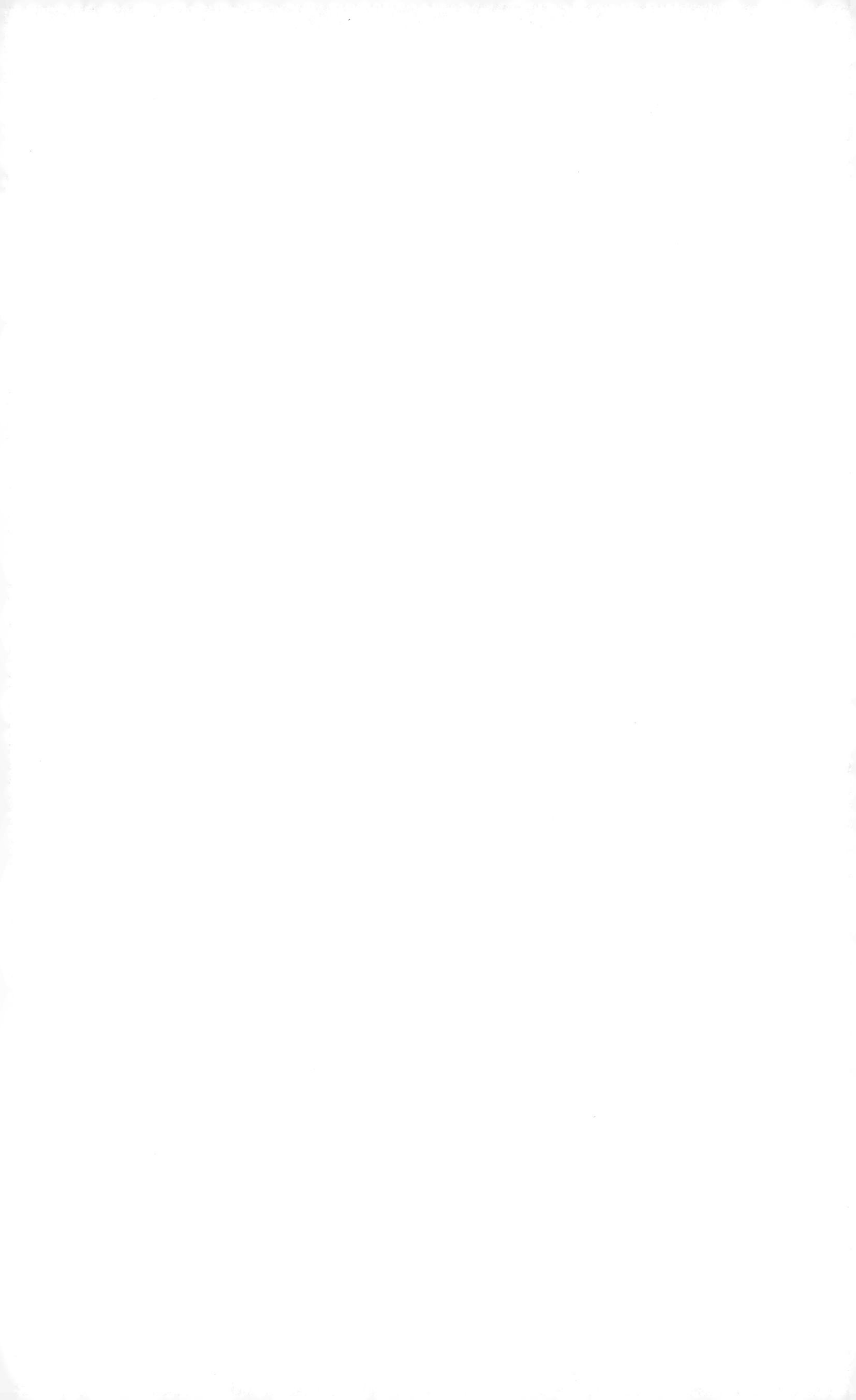

Why I wrote this book...

I decided to write this book because I wish there had been a book like this for me to read when I was considering nursing school. I desperately wanted to have a realistic, detailed idea of what exactly I would be facing and what was involved.

I want to apologize up front from my woeful writing skills. As much as I love to read, I know I'm not a writer. I won't pretend that this is a great work of literature, so please forgive my errors and appalling writing style. My heart is in the right place, so I hope you will forgive the rest.

Everything in this book is from my point of view, based on my first hand experiences. This book is based on completing an ADN RN program so when I say 'nurse" in the text of this book, I'm referring to registered nurse. I'm not insisting that what I'm writing is gospel, but it is the truth of my experience. Your experiences may be much different, but at least you will have a point of reference for your experience and hopefully feel like you are going into these unknown situations with a bit more insight.

I hope that the info in this book will be helpful to all those considering a career in nursing, and help you make more informed choices and help you feel more confident while on this extraordinary journey called Nursing School.

How can you find out if nursing is right for you?

I knew that going back to school to pursue a nursing degree would require a huge investment in time, effort and eventually money (to pay back student loans). I didn't want to find out it wasn't for me half way thru the process.

I decided that the best way to find out if nursing would be right for me, would be to research what nurses had to say about being a nurse. So I tried to get my hands on anything and everything that was written by nurses about what it is like to be a nurse.

So I immersed myself in all the written experiences of nurses that I could find. What I read was at times inspiring; at times hilarious, at times heart-breaking and at times absolutely, disgustingly revolting and I loved it.

As I read, I was waiting to read that one thing that would absolutely turn me off to nursing, but that never happened. In fact, I found myself more and more fascinated by the world of nursing.

But, as my grandmother used to say, "There are a lot of ways to skin a cat." You could also volunteer at a hospital or apply for a CNA (certified nurse assistant). A lot of hospitals have training programs for CNAs or nursing assistants. As a CNA or NA you will see the work nurses do up close. A lot of students in my class worked as CNAs while in school. This also, in some cases, gave them an advantage when it came to landing that first nursing job.

Another great resource is this web site: allnurses.com. It is a site devoted entirely to nurses. Nurses from all over the country and even from other countries post on this site. There is even a forum for student nurses, and just about every nursing specialty. I recommend that you go to the general discussion board, this is were you will find nurses sharing their work experiences and getting feed back from their peers. It is very informative. On this board, nurses will discuss what they love and hate about being a nurse. They will give each other support or debate various topics regarding this profession called nursing. It's a great way to get an 'inside feel' for the world of nursing.

So, how hard is it?

If you tell people you are considering nursing school, it seems that everyone has an idea what its like, based on a friend of a friend's experience. Inevitable they all say it's VERY hard, VERY competitive, the instructors are VERY mean and VERY few people make it through to graduation.

I want to separate the fact from the fiction, and the reality from the horror stories that seemed to be designed to frighten wanna be nursing student into reconsidering their career goals. You should also know that those who have the most harrowing tales of nursing school are those who failed out of their programs.

Is it hard? Yes, it's very hard, but it's doable; the millions of working nurses out there are proof that it can be done.

Remember when I said that nursing school is a journey? Well, it really is like a journey. A crazy ride that goes at times at breakneck speed, and the challenge is to keep up.

At the beginning of every semester, I always felt like I was on a roller-coaster that was perched at the top most peak of a vertical drop. I was tense with anticipation. I knew that once the semester began there would be instant unstoppable momentum and the challenge I would face would be to keep up and not get overwhelmed.

The secret is to prepare. Like any journey, if you have an idea where you are going and what hardship and pitfalls you will face along the way, you can plan in advance and not be taken by surprise and become a victim to circumstance.

The number one, most important thing that you can do to assure you success in nursing school is read your textbook. I know that might seem insulting simplistic, but not when you consider the huge volume of reading that is required of nursing students. Just doing the reading is an awesome accomplishment. Remember that most nursing textbooks weigh ten pounds and are usually 3 inches thick and you will have to read almost all of it.

The real challenge will be finding TIME to accomplish all the reading that you need to do. Here are some strategies that can help you do it.

Find out what modules will be covered in your upcoming semester. You can ask the instructor for this info, and some will happily oblige you and give you this info. From the list of modules and the objectives to be accomplished in each module, you will be able to figure out which chapters of you text you need to read.

What if the instructor won't give you the info? You can ask a student who is currently taking that course. Most students are happily to share this with you. Another thing you can do, is just google the course name and the curriculum requirements for the course will usually come up in the search (if this doesn't work, go to your state board of nursing web site and do a search.). The course requirements are set by your state board of nursing, not your instructor. It's not secret information that you are not allowed to be privy to, no matter how much an instructor would like you to think it is.

As I said, you can use this to figure out what you need to read. I always tried to do all my reading during the breaks between semesters. I know what you are thinking, won't I forget everything if I do my reading so far in advance? Interestingly enough, no. First of all, reading the chapter will give you a first introduction to the material. It will make you familiar with it, you won't actually learn it at that point. It's when your instructor lectures on the material, you will realize that you recall an amazing amount of the material. And not only that, you will be able to ask for clarifications. Clarifications that you would not even know you needed if you had not read the material. Also, the lecture functions as a first review of the material, which means that you leave lecture well on your way to learning the material. At this point, all you have to do is to study and prepare for the exam.

And there is another good reason to do your reading before lecture. There is nothing that nursing instructors seem to hate more than lecturing to a group of slack-jawed, glassy-eyed students whom seem to be completely clueless about the material. They have to prepare their lecture, the least the students can do is prepare for the lecture too. You can actually see the steam pouring out of their ears when they ask the class a question and all they get back are........ crickets.

And then there is always that one student who wants to impress the instructor with their "brilliant, insightful" questions. Questions that they would know the answers to if only they READ THE MATERIAL. This student thinks that they are fooling the instructors but the instructors actually get annoyed because this student is basically asking to be spoon fed, rather than doing the work. They are annoying to other students because they are wasting class time. Don't be that student!

Please trust me and follow my advice. Having your reading done before hand, will be a huge weight off your shoulders and will give you a huge advantage in that you can spend your time studying and getting your other work done. This is nursing school remember, if you don't have your reading done, you will have a mountain of reading to do, and studying, and you probably have to be doing the same for another nursing class and you might have clinicals that week with all the paper work that has to be done for that as well. Quickly, it will seem that the only way to get it all done is find some way to kick the sleeping habit for 3 or 4 days in a row. This is how nursing students get overwhelmed, do badly on exams and eventually flunk out of the program.

Well, what if I just study my lecture notes?
Well, you can try that, but what you will quickly find is that instructors will hold you responsible for everything in the chapter and it is all fair game for the exam wether or not they mentioned it in lecture. And anyway, don't you want to know that the nurse caring for you or your loved one read their nursing textbooks?? I know I do!

Another tip. Use an index card to force yourself to read each and every line before moving on to the next. Unfortunately, most nursing text books aren't exciting page-turners. If you don't find a way to make yourself focus on what you are reading, you will find that though your eyes read the entire page, your brain was composing a list of errands you need to do or rehashing an argument you had earlier with your boyfriend. Index card. It works, I promise!

Yes, there will be math....

Don't panic! The math involved is very basic division and multiplication and addition. The math is related to dosage calculation.

In my program, every semester began with a dosage calculation test. It always felt like the first hoop that we had to jump thru. The lowest passing grade was 90%. Out of 20 problems, we could only miss two, to pass. We were given 3 chances to pass the calculations test. If we failed the 3rd time, it was considered a failure for clinicals, failing clinicals means we failed the semester, and we would not be allowed to continue with the program. Some programs are even tougher when it comes to dosage calculations, giving only one test and requiring the student to get 100% to pass. Make sure you find out your nursing program's policy.

Why so much emphasis on dosage calculations? Medication errors are some of the most serious errors that can have deadly consequences for patients in the health care system. If you or you loved one were hospitalized, you would want to trust that your nurse will give you the correct medication and at the correct dosage, right? Quite literally, a nurse's ability to correctly calculate dosages can mean the difference between life and death for her patients. That is why dosage calculation is such a big deal.

Now that you are throughly freaked out, let me tell you the good news. Dosage calculation is something that you can easily master, if you are willing to put some time and effort into learning how to do it and practice once you learn.

I can't recommend high enough the book Calculate with Confidence. The book can be purchased from amazon and may also be available at your college book store.

If math is one of those subjects that makes your stomach churn, I recommend that you get your trembling, sweaty hands on this book and complete it well before you start your first semester of nursing courses. A chapter can be completed well within an hour and there is a post test you can complete, to assure that you grasp the chapter concepts before moving on to the next. There are two methods given for completing the problems: ratio and proportion and the formula method.
In the first part of the chapter, practice problems are worked out, step by step in each method. Inevitably one of these methods will feel more comfortable to you. That is the method that you can use to work out most problems.

This book also comes with a CD that has hundred of practice problems, but if you buy your book second hand and it doesn't have the CD, just google "dosage calculation practice". You will find many sites you can go to hone your dosage calculation skills.

Failing out of nursing school due to failing the calculations test is something you won't have to worry about, if you put in the time and effort to prevent it.

Creating a study technique that works for you

So, you have your reading done, you went to lecture prepared. You asked the instructor for the clarifications you needed, the next time you show up for this class, it will be to take the exam.

Now you need to study. In order to study effectively, you have to understand the nature of exams in nursing school.

First of all, you will be expected to utilize Critical Thinking. Critical thinking is the ability to correctly apply what you have learned in real world scenarios. The usual format for nursing exams is multiple choice. This is not by accident. Most of the question that you will encounter of the NCLEX exam (National Council Licensure Examination) will be multiple choice, so most of your exams questions in nursing school will be in that format to give you plenty of exposure to this type of question.

Many times, you will find that there will be more that one answer that seems correct. It is up to you to apply what you have learned to determine which answer is correct based on all the factors that must be considered.

The scenarios presented to you on an exam will determine if you understand:
-the nature of a patient's condition
-What conditions the patient is at risk for due to their condition?

-What are the assessments you should make as a nurse, in what order should they be made?
-What are the interventions you the nurse can take?
-What are the medications that may be prescribed?
-What are the potential side effects or contraindications of those medications?
-What is NOT appropriate/correct related to the nursing care of this patient?

When you consider that a module can contain a huge amount of material, the scenarios that it can be applied to it is equally huge. The only way to get yourself into the critical thinking mode and practice applying what you have learned, is to answer and review as many multiple choice/nclex style questions as possible.

Many text books come with a CD that has practice exam questions. There are also review books that you can use. Two of my favorites were Prentice Hall Nursing Reviews & Rationales and Lippincott's Q&A for NCLEX-RN.

What you will find is that after you do a lot of these review questions, is that you will begin to really grasp the concepts presented in the module as they relate to the practice of nursing and what is your role, as the nurse, in the care of those patients. For the questions you answer incorrectly, rationales are provided that explain why that answer is incorrect and why another answer is correct.

Another great resource is evolve.com. You can get the free resources that correspond to your textbook on this web site. These free resources frequently include nclex style questions and a list of glossary terms for each chapter.

I always did at least 100-200 practice question before an exam. Doing this number of question assured that I had covered most all aspects of the module topic.

Prentice Hall Nursing Reviews & Rationales is helpful in another way in that the material that you read in detail in your text is presented in a concise outline format. This makes reviewing a whole module and all the relevant points easier and anything that you aren't sure of can be quickly found and reviewed.

And finally, I have left the best for last. This is an AWESOME web site: quizlet.com. You can search based on module or topic, and you will find a wealth of information. You can create sets of your own, by inputting terms and searching for the list of definitions that are most relevant to you, or input your own. After creating a set, you can have quizet, create a multiple choice quiz using those terms. It is a wonderful resource. Please, check it out!

fellow students

Your fellow students will be a huge source of support for you. They will be the only ones who will understand what you are going thru once nursing school takes over your life.
The experience of going thru nursing school is extraordinary. It will come to dominate and dictate so many aspects of your life. Family and friends may not understand, and you may feel hard pressed to explain how much effort is required to fulfill all the work and why you are so exhausted and stress out by that effort.

In the first semester especially, when everyone is trying to get their bearing and figure out exactly what is expected of them, you will find that you are a great source of support for one another. You will help keep each other on track, you can quiz each other, remind each other of assignment due dates, share what you learned in clinicals, share lecture notes, get clarifications. Share nursing school gossip (what a student currently in the semester ahead had to say about instructor so and so and what a nightmare her/his exams are).

Your classmates will not judge you for being fuzzing on any detail. They know all too well the massive amount of work that is weighing on each of you. They are the ones you can vent to, you can cry on their shoulder. You will encourage each other when you are feeling down and discouraged.

You will probably find that your class is made up of men and women from very diverse backgrounds. You will have some students fresh out of high school and others in late midlife, who are changing careers and everything in between. Though you may all come from different back grounds you will all in time find that nursing school has a way of bonding you together.

At times it will seem like it's the students against the instructors. Right off the bat, many instructors will be very tough. They will very quickly convey to you how seriously they take this business of nursing and they expect you to approach it with the same gravity. It can be very intimidating and it may feel that they are being excessively 'mean' or intentionally trying to weed out the current crop of nursing students.

Every semester, you will see classmates struggle. This is what you can do to help: share study notes, share resources and website that are helpful. But in the end, it all comes down to the individual. They have to take and pass the exam on their own.

It's hard to see a classmate you really like in distress because they know they are failing a class. It's something I promise you will encounter.

You will have to accept that what you can do for them is limited. To successfully complete a course, you must master the modules as they are presented so you can pass the exams and have enough mastery of all the modules to pass the comprehensive final exam. That is the only way to make it thru. You cannot make it thru nursing school on the coat tails of fellow students. Everyone must do their own work.

It's very sad to see someone who has bombed the first three exams and who hangs all hope on 'Acing' the remaining exams and the final to pass the course. Inevitably, this person will not be there for the first day of class for the next semester. It's always sad to realized a classmate has failed the last semester. Of our 52 students that started first semester together, only 18 of us 'ORIGINALS' graduated together.

You will meet a lot of great people in nursing school. These are folks you will always feel fondness for not only because you shared the experience of nursing school together but also because it is a fact, that the field of nursing attracts the some of the most wonderful caring people you will ever meet.

Okay. Now that I've got you feeling all warm and cozy, I have to talk briefly about the other not so great fellow classmates.

A very interesting thing happens right around your 3rd semester. Everything starts to come together. All that pathophysiology and nursing theory that it seem to only exist to torture nursing student, starts to come alive. You start to see what you have learned in the classroom, in your clinical patients.

You begin to understand and put together what your role is as a nurse in the delivery to health care to the patient. You begin to embrace your function within a mult-disincplinary health care system. It all begins to crystalize, and the harsh, critical eye that your clinical instructor used to assess your progression as a student nurse, you internalize and become your own internal critic. You assess your own skills and understanding and begin to measure yourself against the seasoned competent nurses you get the chance to work with.

You also begin to look on your fellow classmates as potential co-workers or colleagues. You may be dismayed to realize that there are some of your classmates that you would not want to work with. Someone who is chronically late, unprepared, they always need help but never have any time to help you. And my all time personal pet peeve: they are unwilling to give up their social lives, so they beg you to do a marathon cram session with them on sunday for the monday morning exam. They tend to make excessive demands of their classmates because they are unwilling to shoulder the lion share of the demands of nursing school themselves.

It's experiences like these that bring home to you a hard cold fact: not everyone who wants to be a nurse, SHOULD be a nurse.

Awwww!!!......nursing instructors!!!

I was late for my very first nursing class.
Ms. R's eyes were like two blue lasers searing into my head as I tried to surreptitiously slink into class and quickly find a seat.
(By the way, that was the first and last time I was ever late for her class.)

She could deliver a lengthy, complex lecture while rare glancing at her notes. She quickly and succinctly answered worthy questions, and dismissed what she deemed as silly or stupid questions with sarcasm and annoyance.

At times she seemed so disgusted with our incompetence that she seemed on the verge of being physically ill. (A few months later, it became apparent that Ms. K was expecting, so perhaps we weren't totally responsible for making her want to hurl.)

You quickly learned that you had to at least have clue about the lecture material before you would dare ask her a question. Many times, she would answer a question, by rapid firing questions right back at you. If you knew the material and the nursing process, she could lead you to the answer to your question.

As uncomfortable as this was, she was trying to get us to apply critical thinking to figure out the answer. This is a vital skill for nurses to have, but to many of us, at the time she just seemed mean and intimidating.

Nursing instructors have a reputation for being very tough and some are. When you consider that they are training you to have the ability to maintain a vulnerable, sick patients' safety, you realize that this training can mean the difference between life and death. They take the job of preparing you for that role very seriously. When you are faced with a situation that requires immediate action on your part to save your patients' life, you will be grateful for an instructor who made sure you were well prepared for that moment.

You will have a lot of different instructors during nursing school and they will all have a different teaching styles. They will also have their own set of pet peeves when it comes to the profession of nursing. As you attend their lectures, you will begin to get an idea of what they think makes a good and competent nurse. These ideas you will also see reflected in their exam questions. This makes having the same instructor for a class helpful. Usually, a new instructor is kind of like an unknown quantity until you take the first exam. After the first exam, you have insight into how they think and what they expect from their students.

Once you take the exam, and put that together with how they lecture, you can begin to understanding of how the instructor "thinks" as a nurse. This helps because you begin to view the information though the prism of the instructors mind set. One instructor may stress pathophysiology, another may stress strict adherence to the nursing process etc..

This is a subtle process, but one you will become aware of as the semester progresses and you get to know your instructor and understand what she expects from you as a nursing student. You will REALLY appreciate this when you have a course taught by several different instructors. You will feel like you are starting all over trying to figure out what each new instructor wants. It can be really stressful.

Finally, please remember that nursing instructors are human and they are affected by the stress that their students are going thru, though they may seem to be aloof. They may come to class in a bad mood, because they just had to tell a student that they were out of the program, while the student tearfully tell them that they are dashing their "dream" to be a nurse. From the instructor's point of view the student dashed their own dreams by not meeting the requirements to earn a passing grade.

Most nursing instructors want to see hard working dedicated students succeed. If you prove to your instructors that you are serious about nursing school you will find that most instructors will try to help you when and if they can (for instance, if you have to miss a clinical due to illness, they might be inclined to cut you some slack and reschedule, than for a student who is chronically late and constantly complains loudly about how it's not fair that nursing school is so hard!)

Most of your instructors will be very organized, and spell out clearly what you must accomplish to pass their class. This is good for everybody, there is no or very little confusion and everyone can get on with getting their work done. You will come to LOVE these types of instructors.

And then there are those who give you very little or confusing information. You will feel like you have to tweeze info out of them. This can be very frustrating for you as a student, you will feel like you have to not only master the objectives of the class, but psychically draw it out of the instructor. I don't know why some instructors are like this, perhaps they are just naturally disorganized, but at times it will feel like they are torturing you by not being forthcoming with the info you need from them.

There are a few things you can do in this case. One of the first is to go talk to a student who has already completed the course. They can be a wealth of info and give you a brief synopsis on the class and tell you what you can expect. The next is to make an appointment with the instructor and bring a list of specific questions. That way you have reserved their time and you are not wasting class time. Hopefully you will get most of your questions answered. It's always good to share any info you get with fellow class mates, an unorganized class causes a lot of stress. Students worry that they will miss something: an assignment, a quiz , etc., these small detail that you might miss out on, could be the difference between passing and failing.

And finally, you should spell out in detail you feelings on the instructor's review at the end of the semester. And if you will not be having anymore classes with that instructor you can also go directly to the director of the program and complain. It's unlikely that an instructor will retaliate against you for complaining, but you can't expect to be one of their favorite students after you do. It may be too late for your class, but hopefully your efforts can make life a little bit better for future students and remember, the school isn't just doing us a favor by letting us be in the program we have worked hard to qualify for the program and we are paying for it. Therefore we have the right to state our concerns.

Finally, I just want to mention my favorite instructor Ms. K. She could be stern and tough, and impatient with students who didn't meet the high standards she set for them. Like a mother hen, she would remind us continually of upcoming assignments. Not all instructors would do this, but she showed that she understood the huge stress and demands we were under as nursing students. It was one way that showed how much she cared for her students.

She could also be very funny. She cracked up the whole class on more times than I can count. I will never forget how she was near tears telling about a young AIDS patient she cared for, and then in the next moment she was composed and continued with lecture. She knew nursing like the back of her hand. When she was please with your work, it felt like the highest compliment. She was an excellent nurse and she had the ability to make you want to be an excellent nurse too.

Thank you for everything Ms. K!

to 'B' or not to 'B'...

A 'C' is the lowest possible passing grade in nursing school. In fact, there is a saying among nursing students, "A 'C' is just as good as an 'A' ". A 'C' student gets the same degree as an 'A' student. So, even a 'C' student can be a registered nurse? So that doesn't seem so hard, right??

Well, it's not that simple. First of all you have to apply the nursing school curve. What that means if that if you are an 'A' student in your general ed classes, you can expect to be a 'B' student in nursing school. If you are a 'B' student in your general ed classes, you can expect to be a 'C' student in nursing school. If you are a 'C' student in your general ed classes, well.... Good luck, nursing school will be a real challenge for you. First of all, you will just barely have a GPA high enough to qualify for most programs and you will have to work hard to maintain it.

So as you can deduce, nursing school usually deals a hit to your GPA. You may enter the program with the GPA equivalent of an 'A' but finish the program with a 'B'. I'm not saying that making an A in a nursing course is impossible, but it is very difficult, and making an A in every nursing course is almost impossible.

In each semester, I always strived for an A on every exam, but I was also satisfied with a 'B'. Maintaining a 'B' average meant that I still had a cushion in the event that I just did really poorly on an exam.

If a student has a 'C' average on the first two exams, they are already on the razor edge. They have to hope that they continue to pull 'C's or do better. If they really bomb the third exam, they may have to make an 'A' to pull their semester average back up to an acceptable level. Remember, most programs require you maintain at least a 'C' in your nursing courses.

This is why maintaining a 'B' average is so important. And the key to doing that is reading and preparation as I have already mentioned. Also a 'B' average can give you what passes for peace of mind in nursing school, otherwise you will be a nervous wreck for 16 weeks and every exam will be a gut wrenching experience.

I can tell you that it is wise to prepare and expect that you might do badly on an exam, despite all efforts. I can recall that there were 3 exams that just seems to come out of left field. In each case, most of the students did poorly on the exam, even those who usually get good grades. In these cases, the instructor formulated oddly worded or confusing questions, or they required nit-picky obscure info, when most students prepare by getting a generalized understanding of a huge amount of material.

I and my fellow students were at a loss to explain these exams. The best we could figure is that the instructor must have temporarily become unhinged while creating the exam.

Crazy, weird, horrible exam. It happens. Don't let it derail you. Get yourself into the mindset, where you only accept a 'B' from yourself. You'll be glad you did.

More exam taking tips:

Turn off your cell phone.
Most instructors will fail you if they hear your cell phone ring or vibrate during an exam. Some even go so far as to take up all cell phones before passing out the exam. It's also a good idea to turn off your cell phone, or at least putting it on vibrate during lecture. Instructors HATE ringing cell phones during lecture. (BTW another great way to make sure your instructor hates you, is to text during lecture or doing Facebook on your lap top during class.)

NEVER, EVER, EVER, change your answers on the exam. If you do, inevitably you will change a correct answer into an incorrect answer. I know lot of you won't believe me on this and will have to learn this lesson first hand, but the chances are always highest that your first answer is correct even if you are not 100% sure. Let the odds work for you! Don't change your answers. The ONLY exception to this rule is if you realize that you misread the question the first time.

Bring at least one extra sharpened pencil. Talking during the exam, even if you are only asking to borrow a pencil, is an automatic failure.

Ask your instructor if you are allowed to write on the exam booklet. If you are, this does give you some advantages. First of all, write your name on your test booklet. Circle each of your answers in the test booklet, but DON'T FORGET TO ALSO MARK THE ANSWER

ON YOUR SCAN-TRON. Even if you circle the correct answer on the test booklet, if it's not on the scan-tron you won't get credit.

Lay your test booklet over your scan-tron, with only the answer number you are currently working on the scantron showing, then move the test booklet down as you work. This prevents you from putting the answer to question 2 in the place for question 3. If you do, all the answers will be skewed and the scantron grading machine will mark them all wrong.

If you don't know an answer, just go with your 'best guess' and mark a small dot next to that question on the test booklet. When you finish the test, go back and count all your 'best guess' questions. If you prepared well for the exam, you will probably get a third to one half of these questions correct. Subtract one half of your best guess answers from the total number, this should be very close to your highest possible score. Subtract two-thirds of your best guess answers from the total number and this should be your lowest possible score. Your actual score should fall somewhere within this range.

This is what I always did, so that I had a good idea of what my grade was at the end of the exam.This is my own highly unscientific method to figure out my grade, I hope it works for you too, but I can't guarantee it.

If you are allowed to write on the test booklet, underline any words like, ‘not’, ‘except’, ‘does not apply’. It is very easy to skip over the word ‘not’ when you are in high tension exam mode.

ex. the nurse knows it is not appropriate to place the patient in respiratory distress in

A. high fowlers (this answer is INCORRECT because it IS appropriate)

B. trendelenburg (this answer is CORRECT because it IS NOT appropriate)

See what a difference the little word 'not' makes? When I was in nursing school, I hated these types of questions. It felt like the instructor was screwing with my head and intentionally trying to cause me to miss the question. But there is a method to this madness. As a practicing RN, the overwhelming majority of instructions you receive related to the care of your patients is in written form. It is of paramount importance that you read what the written material actually says, not what you think it says. These types of questions as infuriating as they are, actually do teach you a valuable skill.

When it comes to exams in nursing school, either you know the answer or you don't. If you understand the nursing process and have a good grasp of nursing interventions, you can usually make a very good educated guess. Skipping over the question, and then going back and staring at the question for twenty minutes, will not make the answer magically come to you. Do your best guess and move on. Don't let yourself get bogged down on any one question. That is my advice.

Usually exams are between 50-100 questions long and usually an hour is allowed to take them some times a little longer. It works out that you are usually allotted one to two minutes per question. Obviously, the fewer questions, the more critical each question is for your grade. The majority of students never come close to needing the whole time allotted to take an exam. Folks who need the whole allotted time usually do poorly.

Some instructors will review the exam after everyone has completed it. If you were allowed to write on the exams, they may pass out the test booklets again. If you wrote your name on yours, you now have a record of all your answers and at the end of the review you will know your score. I was always surprised at the number of student who failed to write their name on the test booklet, so during the review the had to try to remember exactly what their answers were.

Some instructors will allow you to ask questions, after or during the review. Specifically you may want to argue why you feel that the answer what you chose is correct. Some instructors will do a review, but not allow any questions. They require you to submit any argument you may have in written form and site page number of your text that supports my argument. I did this twice and each time, successfully got credit for my answer (woo hoo!!).

Another, really important point i'd like to make is to never miss an exam. Even if you are sick as a dog, I recommend that you drag yourself to class take the exam, you can always leave afterwards and get a fellow student to email you their lecture notes.

Why? Well, some instructors may let you reschedule the exam at a time convenient for you, but most won't. Most will make you take the makeup exam on the day of the final. This means you will have to prepare for the comprehensive final (and most of them are) AND another exam. It may be weeks or months since the lecture when you went over the material. The exams are HARD ENOUGH when the material is fresh in your mind! So why but yourself in the position of having to study for two exams at once? By doing that, rather than doing well on one you may end up just doing so-so on both, or even worse, bombing on one?

And then there is the old assertion that the instructors make the makeup up exam really hard to punish students who miss the exam. I never missed an exam, so I have no first hand knowledge of this and I can't certify that an instructor might not enjoy extracting a little pay back on a student that they feels shows less that proper respect for the instructors time. But I'm inclined to think that a make up exam seems a lot harder, than it would be it if was taken when the material was fresher in your mind.

At the end of every semester there was always some poor sap, bemoaning the fact that they have to take one or two (Ack!) Make up exams on the same day as the final. Nursing school is hard enough, why stack the deck against yourself and make it even harder??

There are different ways that your final grade can be determined. Some instructors assign equal value to the exams and the final (so lets say you have 6 exams and the final exam. Add all you scores together, to get your total points. Divide your total points, by the total possible points : 651/700 = 0.93 = 93% = A (Congrats!))

Then there are times when you exams will be a percentage of your grade and you final will be a percentage. Those percentage are added together to make up your final grade for the course.

Ex. you get 70% of your exam points. Exam points 530/600 x 0.7 = 62. You get 30% of your final exam grade. 68/75 x 0.3 = 27; 62 + 27 = 89% = B (Well done!)

Finally, how will you know you are ready for the exam? Well, this is how I knew I was ready. I had spent so much time studying and going over and over the material and answering nclex questions that I was usually totally and thoroughly sick of the material and ready to move on to something new. I always showed up on exam day, wanting to take it and get it over with. I found that the anticipation of taking the exam was always worse that actually taking the exam.

Clinicals: what to do, what not to do and getting past fear.

First of all these are the things you will absolutely need:

Uniform

There will be weeks when you have more that one clinicals in a week, so 2 uniforms will save you from doing laundry. It's a good idea to have a back up. There is usually someone who had graduated who is more that happy to sell there uniforms. Check around for flyers. This is a great way to save some extra money. My uniform was a flimsy twill, so I bought two white knit tops to wear under them for warmth and keep my bra from showing thru.

Nursing shoes

Some instructors insist on real nursing shoes, some are fine with clean, all white athletic shoes. Find out what is acceptable from your instructors and nursing students who have already done clinicals.

ID badge

Your school will furnish you with this. You can be absolutely prepared in every way for your clinical day, but without your ID you will be dismissed. Your ID lets all the other hospital personnel and patients know who you are and that you have a legitimate reason to be in the hospital. This is a hospital, their first priority is the safety and security of their patients, not providing you with an educational experience. Your ID is your key to the hospital or any clinical setting. DON'T FORGET IT!!

Stethoscope
My advice is to go with something affordable and you can hint that you'd like a Lipman in your choice of color for a graduation present. Amazon has a great selection.

Watch with a second hand
I love my scrub watch. It is all plastic so it can be cleaned with alcohol pads, it also has the military time on it so I know my notation of time on my paperwork is accurate. This watch is available on Amazon.

Pen lights
They come in a pack, make sure you always have one with you, at some point, your clinical instructor will ask you for it, trust me. Not having your equipment, means you made be failed in one of you clinical objectives. You can get them on Amazon.

Bandage Scissors
These are used for dressing changes, opening packaging, I'll guarantee that a clinical instructor will at some point ask for your bandage scissors, don't be without them.

Black pens
Bring more that one, they must be black, not blue and never red! In nursing school, you will be amazed at how quickly pens seem to run out of ink, make sure you always have a good supply. It's not a bad idea to stash them someplace where your kids, husband etc can't get their hands on them. If they know where you keep you

pens, rather looking for one when they need it, they will just take one from your supply and before you know it, you are the one desperately searching for a black pen. Take my advice and hide them!

Alcohol Pads

You can purchase these at any pharmacy. You will mostly use them for cleaning your stethoscope. By doing this you are preventing the transfer of pathologic microorganisms from patient to patient or from patient to yourself, via your stethoscope. Also, it only works to your benefit for your clinical instructor to see you taking steps to protect your patients and yourself and sets a good example for your fellow students.

Appearance

If your hair is long enough to touch your shoulders, it should be neatly pulled back. Make-up should be minimal and natural looking. Visible tattoos should be covered if possible. All piercings should be removed. One set of simple post earrings is usually okay, but no hoops or dangly earrings.

Your uniform should look neat. If you neatly fold it when it comes out of the dryer, you won't have to iron it.

We were told that we could be dismissed from clinicals if our clinical instructor thought we looked unprofessional or disheveled. So please, make sure your uniformed doesn't look like you slept in it.

Your nails should be clean, and short, clear, unchipped polish is usually acceptable. No colored polish or acrylic nails. No dragon lady finger nails, even if they are natural and unpolished.

No strong perfumes, or strongly perfumed soaps. Remember you will be around a lot of sick people who can be especially sensitive to smells. Post-op patients can have nausea related to after effects of anesthesia, strong smells can make it even worse.

And do not under any circumstance allow yourself or your uniform to smell like cigarette smoke. After one whiff, most clinical instructors will dismiss you from clinical.

You may feel that these rules are too restrictive and you might be miffed to find that the nursing staff in the hospital or at your clinical site don't adhere to these guidelines, but as employee, their dress code and appearance is set by their facility and enforced by their manager. You are not an employee, but a nursing student, and as such, you will the expected to have a humble, but professional appearance and attitude. The thing that should set you apart and make you stand out in clinicals should be your professional demeanor, your preparation for the clinical and your enthusiasm for learning what the clinical experience has to teach you.

You must know the ABCs

Every nurse (and health care professional for that matter) knows the rule for priority assessment: ABC. In order to even begin functioning competently in the clinical setting you must live and breath the ABC's. It must be the prism through which you view each and every clinical scenario.

A: stands for Airway. Airway is ALWAYS your first priority. Without an airway, your patient will die. Without an airway everything else you do for your patient won't matter. When assessing a patient, airway is always first.

B: stands for Breathing. Breathing is ALWAYS your second priority (see why airway is first? Without a patent (open) airway, breathing is not possible). Once you know the patient has an airway, you must determine if they are breathing. If they are breathing, is it adequate? (You will also learn that certain patterns of breathing can clue you in to what is going on with your patient.) Inadequate breathing (ventilation) can rapidly cause PH imbalances that damage tissues and eventually can be incompatible with life. If they aren't breathing, you must ventilate them with an ambu bag, till a doctor can intubate them.

C: stands for Circulation. The whole purpose of breathing is to delivery oxygen to tissues and remove carbon dioxide from the tissues. Most importantly, the brain and heart must receive adequate circulation (perfusion). Without adequate circulation, damage to the brain and heart can quickly occur and present a dismal outlook for the patient.

Imagine you are an ER nurse, two patients arrive at your ER at the same time. One is bleeding profusely and screaming. The other is choking and gasping for breath. Which patient do you attend to first? That's right. The choking patient, who clearly seems to have an obstruction in their airway. The screaming patient clearly has a patent airway and is breathing.

The Do's and Don'ts to surviving clinicals

Do always follow Universal Precautions

You must protect yourself and the patients that you come in contact with from pathologic microorganisms (bacteria, viruses, fungi, or parasites that are capable of producing illness of disease).

The best way to do this, is using universal precautions. The main principle is to AWAYS assume that ALL body fluids that you might be exposed to are infectious, and take steps to avoid direct contact with these fluids. In most cases, this will mean wearing gloves, but in other cases it will mean wearing a gown, mask, gloves and goggles. You will come to anticipate what types of contact you must protect your self from (airborne, contact, droplet , etc.) and the types of PPE (Personal Protective Equipment: gloves, gown, mask etc.) required.

It is always a good idea to wipe off all surfaces you will come in contact with in you patients' room and your work station at the beginning of your shift. If you weren't a germa-phobe before nursing school, you will be one after. The nasty virulent bugs out there and the devastation they wreak will give you a whole new awareness.

There are even some nurses who are so concerned about inadvertently bring these bugs into their homes that they change clothes at work, or in their garages and never wear their nursing shoes inside their homes for fear that a family member might contract a bug that is clinging to their scrubs or shoes.

Finally, as a wise nursing instructor once said to me, the first thing you should do for your patient on entering their room is WASH YOUR HANDS!

Don't lose your equipment

Clinical instructors rarely come to clinicals with clinical equipment. If they need a stethoscope, they will ask you for yours. This is something they do to assess your preparedness for clinical. Make sure that you always retrieve your equipment. The instructor may get caught up in her instruction and may set your stethoscope to the side or even drape it around her neck out of habit. Remember to get your stuff back! You don't want to run around the unit trying to find your stethoscope. If a fellow student borrows something from you (Get it together pal!), ask that they return it asap. You don't want your clinical instructor to ask you for your pen light and you have to explain that you don't have it because you loaned it to a fellow student. This just make you both pathetic in the eyes of your instructor.

Do get a good night's rest

Try to get a good nights sleep the night before clinical. This can be difficult at times and almost everyone has pulled an all-nighter trying to complete pre-clinical paper work. Especially at the start of a new semester and you have a new clinical instructor and you are getting used to new paperwork requirement.

Don't party the night before clinical

So staying up all night, to prepare for a clinical is expected, but staying up all night to go to a bachelor/ette party is unacceptable. A clinical instructor can excuse you from clinical even if she just suspects you might be hung-over and not in a fit condition to care for patients. And don't think you can fool them. Clinical instructors are in most cases, seasoned nurses who have seen it all, they can spot a hangover with their eyes closed. Being excused from clinical would result in a failure, a failure in clinical means you cannot pass the semester.

Don't say you don't want to provide a certain type of care

Do yourself a favor and never, ever, say something that sounds even remotely like you don't want to deal with poop, within earshot of your clinical instructor. A resourceful clinical instructor will find you an assignment that will assure that you will spend the next 6 hours of your life dealing exclusively with massive amounts of poop. The lesson is that we don't pick and choose what types of care we give our patients. We give them the care that they require, whatever that may be.

Do give yourself plenty of extra time to get to your clinical site.

You must be at the hospital at 6am. You live twenty minutes from the hospital, so you just need to leave your house by 5:30 am, right? WRONG!

The first thing that you must remember that once your get to the general/visitor parking of the hospital, it will take you at least ten minutes to get to the unit where your clinical is. And that's when you get a prime parking spot, know how to navigate the miles of hospital corridors without getting lost and have minimal to no wait for elevators. But you are a nursing student, so you should expect that the parking area that you are assigned is in the farthest corner, of the farthest parking lot that is still technically on hospital property.

You will need to give yourself at least fifteen minutes to get to your clinical site, once you park. Your clinical instructor will be there usually a little before the start of the clinical day. As each student arrives, your instructor will note the time. One minute past 6am means you are late and will earn you an F in professionalism.

Don't try to park where you not supposed to

If you are assigned a particular place to park, park there and only there. Those unattractive, identical nursing school uniforms make it very easy to an eagled-eye clinical instructor spot you parking in the visitor parking near the hospital entrance. (The uniform also makes it easy for them to spot a gaggle of their students who have slipped away to the front entrance of the hospital for a smoking break.) You may think you have gotten away with this till your instructor makes note of it on your clinical evaluation and failed you in your professionalism objective

.

Don't let your instructor see you checking your cell or god forbid, texting.

It's even better is to turn off your cell all together. The way the clinical instructor sees it, you BELONG to them for the next 6 hours. They expect and demand your undivided attention. If you absolutely must check your phone, (lets say you have a sick kid home with the babysitter) do it in the restroom stall, where you will not be observed or heard. Why? Because the unit nurses will report any unprofessional behavior to your clinical instructor. That's right! It's not just your instructor who is watching you, but the other unit nurses and PCAs as well!

Do report any out of the ordinary occurrence to you clinical instructor ASAP.

If your patient falls, throws up, seems to have trouble swallowing properly, suddenly becomes diaphoretic (sweaty), hyperventilates (>20 breaths a minute), hypo-ventilates (<12 breaths a minute), has syncope (light-headedness with or without fainting), becomes disoriented, intentionally or accidentally pulls out an IV, curses at you, tries to hit you, threatens to hit you, exposes themselves to you, speaks to you in any inappropriate way. Anything and everything that you think might be slightly outside of normal, you should report to your clinical instructor and to your nurse (the unit nurse who is assigned your patient) you must not fail to report any variances to your clinical instructor. Don't even THINK you can hide some occurrence from the nurses or your instructor. The patients talk to their nurses and the nurses will tell your instructor. All of the things I mentioned and more than could ever be listed, are 'normal' variances that occur with patients. Things happen and as a nursing student, you are not Yet equipped or expected to deal with these thing on your own. By reporting these events you are making sure that steps can be taken to assure the patient's safety and that you're nursing career isn't over before it even began.

Don't ever leave your patient's room till....

1) The bed is lowered to the lowest level. Why? If your patient falls while trying to climb out of bed, they are at less risk for serious injury if the bed is set at the lowest level.
2) Make sure the call light/button is within reach of the patient and they know how to use it. Why? What is the number one reason patients try to climb out of bed and end up falling? BINGO! Make sure your patient can summon a nurse without risking life and limb.

Do expect to see some shocking thing

You can count on seeing some wild things during in your clinicals.

The first really bad thing I saw during a clinical, was a truly appalling 4th stage pressure ulcer on a patient who was transferred from a LTC (long term care facility; AKA nursing home).

The patient's sacrum and the spinal nerves that extended from it was clearly visible in the crater-like wound. It was like observing an anatomy dissection, but the patient was still alive. I was shocked and appalled at the level of neglect the patient had had to endure to cause such a terrible condition.

The next, was a patient who was admitted five days earlier with a few necrotic toes. The patient was not aware that they were diabetic and had injured their toes. The injury resulted in infection that quick destroyed the tissue of the toes.

The doctor told the patient that the toes needed to be amputated. The patient refused.

Five days later, more that half of the foot was necrotic. It was black smelled awful and there was foul purulent slough coming out of what was now a hole that went all the way thru the foot. Oh, and the toes the patient didn't want amputated? They had fallen off.

Now the doctors told the patient that the foot needed to be amputated and again the patient refused.

It was distressing to see patient engaging in denial so deep that it could kill them.

I tried to look at the situation and figure out how the patient could be successfully treated and their wish to avoid amputation could be honored but in this case those options were incompatible. Amputation was the ONLY treatment. This was a battle of wills that the patient couldn't win. Not unless they considered dying of overwhelming septic shock winning.

They had come to the hospital, clearly that meant they wanted help. Why were the refusing the only help that could be given? It was a very distressing situation to me on so many levels.

The sight, smell and impact of those experiences have stayed with me. I've seen other situations since that are on par with those, but the FIRST TIME you experience it, it stays with you. You have the same visceral, emotional response that any caring person would have, but then another extraordinary thing happens. You aren't just an ordinary person, you are a nursing student! You are privileged to have the knowledge to do something about these situations. You begin to think like a nurse. Why does the patient have this condition? What will the doctor's treatment plan be? What is my role in carrying out that treatment? What does the patient's condition put them at risk for? (How can this get worse?) What nursing interventions can reduce or eliminate those risks? (What can I do to make sure it doesn't get worse?)

That's right, by the time you get to your senior semester's clinicals, grisly, gruesome injuries will present an intriguing dilemma that will challenge you and make you bring to bear all of your knowledge, to figure out. It is exhilarating when you realize that you have the knowledge to help patients heal.

Don't do anything without your instructors okay

Never do any skill, particularly one that is invasive such as: starting an IV, cauterization, pushing IV meds, blood draws, administering injections, without the express approval of your clinical instructor.

Most instructors are happy to let you practice these skills, but in most cases they will want to observe and supervise. In some cases, they will let you preform a skill with the nurse doing the observation and supervising. Many times you will suddenly get a chance to do a skill, but you have no idea where your instructor is so you can get their okay. It's a lot to ask a busy nurse to wait, while you go track down your instructor. For this reason, it's always a good idea to ask your clinical instructor during the pre-clinical conference if there are any skills that you are not allowed to perform with your nurse.

Do always make sure your handwriting is neat and legible.

You may be required to do the bulk of your clinical paperwork by hand. For this reason it is very important that it is legible. Nothing will make an instructor dread grading your paperwork and as a result unleash scathing criticism on your paperwork, than the headache they will get from squinting and trying to decipher your sloppy scrawl. One of our instructors actually refused to even try to read a set of sloppy paper work and just wrote a gigantic, red '?' across the first page and failed the student for paperwork.

The issue of poor handwriting is one you will become well acquainted with as a nursing student. Just imagine this, there you are on the start of your clinical day. You have been assigned a really interesting patient and are very excited to get started.

As a diligent nursing student, the first thing you do is track down the chart and check for new orders from the patient's doctor. You find the correct page and this is what you see. A series of long dash lines with a few random bumps and squiggles and then more dashes squiggle, squiggle, bump, bump (Oh! That one has a dot above it, it must be an 'I'!) Dash bump, squiggle, bump and it's all finished up with a big squiggle and a long flourishing dash........What the......??

Yep, doctors are notorious for having the worst handwriting. You will be forced to ask a busy nurse to stop what she/he is doing to decipher the gobbledygook for you. It's really annoying. (One unsung skill nurses develop is the ability to decipher a doctor's most obscure goobbledygookish handwriting, bet you didn't know that!) But it's not just doctors, you will find that some nurses have atrocious handwriting too. I remember trying to read a nurse's stylized bubbly, loopy-loopy script. It was impossible.

Obviously, that nurse thought whatever she wrote down was important information about her patient, too bad that no one could actually read it.

Writing something that is illegible is almost as bad as not writing anything at all. And when it comes to nursing, documentation is vitally important. There is a saying, "If your didn't document it, you didn't do it". Writing clearly can save your career and your license. It can prove that you acted in your patient's best interest, rendered the highest standard of care and followed your facility's protocol. It's really is that important. Please get into the habit of writing clearly and legibly.

Do always put your clinical paper work in a folder

Make sure that the folder has your name clearly written on the front and back. Since you have worked so hard on your paperwork, do place your work in a neat, clean folder. This lets your clinical instructor know that you take pride in your work and that you are making it easy and convenient for your instructor to review your work, without getting it mixed up with someone else's.

Don't assume that all elderly folks are hard of hearing

Presbycusis or age related hearing loss affects many older patients. Many, but not all. Unfortunately, since a lot of elderly do have hearing loss, many nurses and PCAs will just automatically raise their voices when speaking to these patients wether or not they know for a fact that these patients suffer from hearing loss.

Once I had a delightful, really interesting patient assignment. The patient was very kind and patient with me, and nursing care involved with the plan of care was very interesting. I was really enjoying taking care of this patient. At one point as we chatted, the patient told me that they liked me better than their assigned nurse, "Because they (the nurse) is always shouting at me."

I realized that the nurse had just assumed that the patient was hard of hearing. This was terribly unfortunate, because the nurse was a wonderful, caring nurse, very competent with lots of experience, but due to a misunderstanding on the part of the nurse, she had inadvertently offended and alienated patient. This assumption the nurse made was clearly having a negative affect on the therapeutic and trusting relationship that should exist between patient and nurse.

When you do have a patient with presbycusis, speak loudly and clearly using simple words. It is also helpful to look directly at the patient because many folks with hearing loss have developed the ability to read lips.

Do check two patient identifiers before administering any medications

Even if you have spent the last five hours getting to know everything and more about Ms. Smith, you must still ask her name, and check her wrist band for her name and birthday or hospital ID number before giving her any medication. That is because the RIGHT PATIENT is the first in the five rights of medication administration. (The 5 rights: the right patient, the right drug, the right dose, the right route, and the right time). Following this protocol will assure that you are always giving the correct meds to the correct patient.

Do make sure that you know all the meds you will be administering during your clinical including PRN meds.

When you do your pre-clinical you will get your patient assignment and have a chance to review you patient's MAR (medication administration record). Write down all the meds your patient is scheduled to receive during your clinical.

You must know the class of drug, why it is given, any contra indications, and the most common side effects. Clinical instructors love quizzing students about medications and they usually do it while you are at the patient's bedside, so it's particularly nerve racking to have your instructor quizzing you and the patient watching you too.

You also need to know if there are any special considerations with a drug. If a drug can be potentially renal toxic, tell your instructor that you know that you need to carefully review the patient's latest labs pertaining to renal function. If a drug requires blood levels to be drawn, tell your instructor that you will check to see what the last labs were. Don't just tell her/him, but go check. Your clinical instructor may follow up at some time and ask you about those labs, you don't want to be caught like a deer in the headlight when and if they do.

Don't ever leave medications unattended.

Your clinical instructor or nurse will remove the meds from the Pyxis (computerized medication dispenser) and then give them to you. You should then go directly to the patient and administer them. Don't set them down on the nursing station while you look around for the glucometer, because you wanted to do the patients's blood sugar when you finish with the meds. A clinical instructor who sees you turn your back on your medication may choose to fail you in medication administration. If all you get is a scolding, consider yourself lucky.

Remember, that many of the drugs we administer in the hospital setting are also controlled substances. You must exercise the utmost care when administering these meds. Unfortunately, addiction and nurse impairment related to drug use is all too common. You should know that if any

narcotics that were in your custody are lost and are not given to the patient, suspicion will fall on you. I don't know what happens in this case. It has never happened in my program. i think it's safe to say that a student in this situation would at the very least be failed for clinicals, and the semester, if not kicked out of the program all together.

Once during my senior semester, I was administering meds at the patient's bedside. I was having trouble trying to open very stubborn blister package. I applied a bit too much muscle causing a Lortab to pop out, become airborne and eventually land on the floor. Mortified (this happened in front of the patient and the patient's nurse), I apologize to the patient and the nurse and told them I would get another tablet. I picked up the tablet and went to my instructor and explain what happened. She, and another nurse as witness, put the tablet down the sink drain in the medication room and turned on the water, so that the tablet was absolutely washed away. This is the process of WASTING. It is always witnessed by another registered nurse and is then documented. It verifies that controlled substances are properly disposed of and there is no hint of suspicion that any nurse is acting improperly and god forbid, taking the medication herself. If for whatever reason a controlled medication is not given to your patient, you must make sure that it is wasted properly and that the wasting is properly witnessed and documented.

Any problems with any of these steps can be devastating to you career.

If you patient refuses a med, or says they will take it later, don't leave the medication at the bedside, instead go explain the situation to your instructor and give the medications to her or the patient's nurse.

If a patient tells you that they don't recognize one of the meds, don't insist that they take it any way, instead, take the medication and double check that it is the correct.

Do ask your clinical instructor for clarification for his/her comments on your paperwork.

Your clinical paperwork should be marked clearly 'pass' or 'fail'. If it is not ask your instructor if you passed or not. If your instructor says you passed, ask them to write that on your paperwork. This is very important because, even though your paperwork may have so much red ink on it that is looks like someone lost most of their blood volume on it, it could still be passing paperwork....Or maybe not.

The following is a cautionary tale that actually happened to me.

I was scheduled to have 3 clinicals with Ms R. Ms. R was like a sphinx. Her facial expression was an enigmatic, unreadable non-expression. She was very soft spoken and spoke very little. She seemed very reserved, with a thin veneer of barely perceptible but unmistakable, harshness. Basically, she was kind of scary and impossible to read.

This can present a problem for nursing students. We tend to gauge our progress from day to day in the non-verbal clues we pick up on from our instructors. Do they seem annoyed with us? Impatient? Disgusted by our incompetence or cluelessness? Or do they seemed pleased? Satisfied? Do they make it clear that they know that you know the answer and wished you'd shut up and give someone else a chance to answer (overwhelmingly the attitude my instructors had toward me! Ha!). This made having Ms. R. for a clinical instructor uncomfortable, but I wasn't too worried about it. I was a hard worker who gave 100% in my clinicals.

The day before my first clinical with Ms. R, I went to the hospital for my pre-clinical. Got my patient assignment, reviewed my patient's chart and gathered all the data I would need to complete my pre-clinical paper work and prepare for my clinical day that would begin the next day at 6am.

On the morning of our first clinical day, Ms. R's instructions where very brief, "Do your assessment". My clinical day went very well. I did my head to toe assessment and filled in all my findings on the clinical assessment sheet that was part of our clinical paperwork for that semester. It was totally complete and neatly done. I reviewed my patient's latest lab work, checked the chart for new orders. I administered all my patient's meds with Ms R. I knew all my meds and answered all the questions she put to me regarding them. I gave my patient a bed bath, changed their linens, took their vitals, assisted my patient

to the bedside commode and kept track of all 'I and o's' (input and output; fluid in, fluid out; how much fluid they drank and IV fluid they received (input), and how much they urinated (output)). I had documented each nursing action I had done in my nursing notes with the time and my signature on each entry. At the end of the clinical I turned in my paperwork neatly arrange in a folder. I was glad to be done with another clinical. I had no worries. I felt I had done well.

A few days later, Ms. K the sections main instructor, handed out the clinical paperwork back to us. Ms. R. had written only one sentence at the top of my nursing notes, "Where is your assessment?" That was it. There were no notes or comments on any other the other pieces of my paperwork.

I was puzzled. There was a huge legal size document clearly labeled "clinical assessment sheet" that I had filled in completely with detailed head to toe assessment findings. What was she talking about? Then I realized that on my nursing notes, I had failed to document that I had done my head to toe assessment. In nursing, if you don't document it, you didn't do it. That must be what she was referring to! She had told me to "do my assessment" and I had failed to document that I had done it. I assumed that the completed assessment sheet would be proof that I had obviously done it. I made a mental note to remember to document doing my assessment in my nursing notes for the next clinical. Which is exactly what I did. Problem solved, right? ....Wrong!

A few days later, Ms. K unexpectedly called me. She wanted to let me know that Ms. R had failed me for the second time on my clinical paperwork. I was shocked! I literally had to sit down, because I felt weak and like I was going to throw up. Two failures! She had not written 'fail' on my first set of paperwork! She had written it on my clinical evaluation sheet though, and the evaluation sheets were not given to us to review the day we were given our graded paperwork, so there was no way for me to know that she had failed me. I asked Ms.K to

Please look at my second set of paperwork (the second set of paperwork had not yet been returned to me) and tell me why she was failing me for a second time. She looked at the paperwork and told me that all Ms. R had written on my second set of paperwork, "No assessment".

I told Ms K I don't understand why she keep saying I have not done my assessment when it is obvious that I had done my assessment. Now I was really upset and starting to hate Ms R, because she had brought me a hair's breadth away from failing the whole semester. I felt like she was capriciously playing with me. She clearly hated me, and I didn't know what in the world I had done to incur her wrath! Since I was so upset, Ms. R said she would call Ms. R and see if she could find out what the problem was.

This was a very serious situation. 3 failures in one objective would mean a failure for clinicals, and failing clinicals means you fail the whole semester. If I failed a semester, I would have to apply for remediation, and have to complete that in one semester, before I would be allowed to re-enter the program and retake the semester I failed. This whole process would put me 6-8 months behind everyone else in my class! I couldn't believe that I was facing this prospect after working so hard.

Finally, Ms. K. called me back. She told me that Ms. R failed me on both sets of paperwork because I didn't included a narrative assessment. Oh.......! I was supposed to know that when she said assessment, she meant a narrative assessment (which is a very specific thing). First of all, doing an assessment is not synonymous with creating a narrative assessment. They are two different things, but that doesn't really matter because.....

One privilege of being a nursing instructor is being vague and obtuse (not all instructors are this way, in fact, most instructors go out of their way to make sure that things are crystal clear and there are no misunderstands when it comes to what is expected of their students) but there are some instructors who seem to enjoy being vague and watching students struggle as a result....ARG!! This makes it the job of every nursing student to ask for clarification. And this is really where I failed.

This is what I should have done:

1) When I got back paperwork that wasn't clearly marked pass or fail. I should have asked the instructor if I had passed and if so to mark it on the paper.

2) I found the instructor's comment puzzling, but tried to figure it out by myself, instead of just asking the instructor to explain exactly what she meant.

3) Finally, if I'm brutally honest, I have to admit that I avoided doing 1 and 2 because I found Ms. R intimidating and kind of scary and I wanted to avoid dealing with her any more than I absolutely had to. Basically, I was chicken, and I paid a price for it.

Needless to say, on my third and final clinical, I wrote out the most amazing, detailed, perfect narrative physical assessment that was ever done in the whole history of nursing school. I passed my paperwork and I passed the semester and learned an important lesson....Whew!

And this naturally leads to the next Do..... Do learn how to write a narrative physical assessment

In nursing school, it seems that there are somethings that you are just expected to learn by osmosis. At times, it seems that the instructors assume that we students will just automatically understand and see the importance of certain concepts. Unfortunately, this is not always the case, but hopefully you will have a wonderful instructor that will teach you something really important that you had no idea you needed to know.

In this case the wonderful instructor I'm referring to is Ms. W. She was hired by my school, because more clinical instructors were needed. It was truly a stroke of luck for my program and I was very lucky to be in the clinical group that was assigned to her, though I didn't realize it at the time. She was a petite Latina, who had an encyclopedic knowledge of nursing theory and process as well as pathophysiology and pharmacology. She knew it all. And I never had an instructor who was more dedicated and passionate about upholding standards of excellence in nursing. She held a masters degree and was a nurse practitioner. She was an excellent mentor.

Our first clinical day with Ms. W went well, but it was in post-clinical conference that we realized that it was not going to be 'business as usual' with Ms. W. She asked us if we where being taught how to take our head to toe assessment data and create a narrative physical assessment. None of us had any idea what she was talking about.

She spent almost an hour explaining what a narrative physical assessment was, why it is important and that she expected us to do one in addition to all of the other paperwork we were expected to do. Inwardly, we all groaned, Great! More work! Thanks Ms. W!

It's completely impossible that she didn't pick up on our less than enthusiastic attitude, but she persisted. She was determined to teach us wether we liked it or not.

As I struggled to learn how to write a NPA (narrative physical assessment), I realized that in my text books there were many examples of narrative assessments. I had read them with interest, but without understanding how important they were. It was a case of not seeing the forest for the trees, till Ms. W came along and pointed out the obvious and made us learn something that was really important. At the end of the semester, we all knew how to take our assessment data and fashion a coherent, complete and polished narrative assessment.

The ability to write a narrative assessment was extremely helpful to me in the following semesters and it will be extremely helpful in your nursing practice. As a practicing nurse your won't be writing out a narrative physical assess, but you will be composing one as you give report at the end of the your shift to the nurse who will take over the care of your patient. If you feel you need to call your patient's doctor, you will need to give him or her an organized, complete narrative assess that clearly lays out why you felt you needed to call them.

Do tell your clinical instructor what skills you have not gotten a chance to do

If you have not gotten a chance to start an IV tell your instructor in pre-clinical conference. She will make sure that the unit nurses know that a student would like to do that skill. You may not get to do every skill you request, but usually between the instructor and the nurses, you will usually get to do and see some interesting things.

Don't forget to ask your instructor and the nurses for feedback

Your instructors and the unit nurses are a 'treasure trove' of information and experience. You will be amazed at the interesting tips, pointers, little tricks that they will share will you if you just get them to start talking. Nurses love talking shop. They will share so much of their knowledge, experience and insights with you if you just show a desire to learn. This is where you will personally experience the generous, giving nature so many nurses process.

And always make sure that you thanks them for sharing these thing with you. They didn't come by their knowledge easily. It is usually the result of years of hard physical and mental work. It's an extraordinary thing that they are happily willing to share with us.

Do challenge yourself in your clinicals

It's really important to take advantage of your clinicals. As a student, you are expected to be terrible and clueless. You will not be expected to do anything well and there will always be either your instructor or an experienced nurse standing by ready to take over if you can't manage something. You can only improve and as long as you try your best and put forth genuine effort to learn, you don't have to worry about disappointing your instructor or the nurses. Your eagerness to learn is what matters.

Don't be a wallflower in clinicals. Don't look for or hope for the easy assignment. Challenge your self! Make inquiries of the unit nurses. Find out who is the most 'challenging' (sickest) patient on the floor. If that patient is not assigned to any other student, ask your instructor if you can be assigned that patient. Your instructor may be impressed that you are asking for a tough assignment, but more importantly, you will learn so much from taking care of that patient. What you learn from them will make you a better nurse.

You will never again have a situation as a nurse, where it will be so safe and beneficial for you to really step outside your comfort zone. There will always be a nurse and your clinical instructor there to guide you and step in when and if things get hairy, so there is no risk to you or to the patient. Once you are a practicing nurse, if you are given an assignment that feels 'really challenging' and is pushing you 'out of your comfort zone', the responsible thing to do is refuse the assignment. If you don't feel confident that you are completely competent to give that patient the level of care they need, you should not agree to care for them. To do otherwise, puts the patient and your license at risk. Take advantage of the unique situation nursing school clinicals offer.

Don't ever tell the patient that you know how they feel

Unless you are laying in the bed next to them with the same medical condition and same prognosis, there is no way that you can know how the patient feels. When a patient complains or vents, the safest and best first response is to say, "I'm sorry....That you are not feeling well." "I'm sorry....That you are upset."etc. The next best thing is to ask them, "Is there is anything that you would like me to do for you?" If they don't have any requests, suggest something that you can do for them. Patients don't need you to understand so much as they need to know you care.

Also another thing you must remember is that as nurse, you are a safe target for the patient's anger and frustration. If they are in pain, or feeling out of control, they can direct this at you. You must strive to be professional. This means not taking it personally. You still have to help the patient even when they are not pleasant. They can yell at you and be nasty to you and not worry about the result. Being nasty to their wife or husband carries a greater risk. They need the love and support of their loved ones. You are paid to do a job, so they don't have to worry about or concern themselves with your feelings.

We are supposed to hold our patients in unconditional positive regard. This doesn't mean we have to love them, but we need to give them the benefit of the doubt and cut them some slack, they are sick after all and dealing with the stress and upheaval of their lives that comes with that.

....And yes, do expect there to be blood, pus, snot, vomit, urine, poop and sometimes.... people will die.

First and most important thing to remember: always treat ALL bodily fluids that you have to deal with as potentially infectious and protect yourself from direct contact with them. Always use gloves and use goggles, mask and gowns when appropriate.

No nurse likes dealing with this stuff, but it comes with the territory. Many of the patients you will encounter in your clinicals are seriously ill, so ill at times, that they cannot attend to their bodily functions. In order to maintain the patient's dignity and protect the patient, this fun job will fall to you.

Keeping your patient clean, keeps their skin intact. Any break in the skin can lead to potential infection. Patients who are already sick, many times have a depressed immune system and their bodies are unable to mount an adequate immune response to an infection, this can lead to life-threatening sepsis.

When it comes to cleaning a patient who is soiled with feces, or as many nurses refer to it, 'a code brown' a registered nurse can delegate this task to a PCA. That is if there is a PCA available to do the task quickly (feces, especially diarrhea, has a lot of enzymes that can quickly begin to breakdown the skin). If there is no PCA available to do it, you must attend to your patient. Do not think that cleaning soiled patients is the only a PCA's job. As the nurse, you are responsible to the care of your patient.

If a family member arrives to visit their loved one and finds them laying in a puddle of excrement. You will be the only one they will yell at. You are the one they will complain to the unit manager about. You are the one your unit manager will yell at. Even though you may have delegated the task to someone else, you must follow up and make sure the task is done properly and in a timely fashion.

A willingness to 'get your hands dirty' (just a figure of speech, please, always wear gloves!) Will let everyone you work with know that you don't set yourself above any nursing task that needs to be done.

Fortunately, as a nursing student, nurses and PCA are happy to let you practice dealing with code browns. Lucky you!

Here are a few tips:

-Buddy up with a fellow student: you help them clean their patient. They help you clean yours. This task really is more manageable with two sets of hands and a person on each side of the bed, the first few times you do it. If your patient is confused, has dementia or any condition that makes them unable to understand that you are trying to help them and co-operate, you should get assistance.

-Gather all the supplies you will need in advance. Make sure you have at least two briefs (Adult diapers, BTW always call them briefs. This shows respect for your patient and maintains their dignity) make sure they are the right size. Before you remove the soiled one, note where on the hip it is placed. If you place it too high on the hip, you will not have enough of the brief in the front to secure it properly and make sure that it won't leak. You might not know what i'm talking about now and have a hard time visualizing it, but once you attempt to put a brief on a patient, you will know exactly what i'm talking about. I promise.

-Have a soiled linen bin outside your patient's room (if the facility doesn't use them, get a soiled linen bag).

-Draw the patient's curtain to provide your patient with privacy.

-Raise the bed, so you can work without straining your back.

-Tell the patient what you are doing and why. Even if you don't think they can hear you or understand, that is besides the point, being respectful to the patient and upholding their dignity is just as important as any nursing care you provide to your patient.

-Double glove your hands: remove the first set of gloves after you have cleaned the feces and removed soiled linen. They are contaminated and you don't want to be touching clean items with them but you still have on a clean set of gloves on to finish up the task.

-If the patient has diarrhea, you should wear a gown to protect your clothes. (If they have been receiving antibiotics, they probably do have diarrhea. If they have C. diff, they will be on contact precautions, it will be posted in their door and the PPE (personal protective equipment) you will need should be on a cart next to their door.

-Wash you hands before you leave the patient's room and afterward use hand sanitizer.

-Try to work quickly and systematically, and don't let the patient get chilled. If they are cold afterward, get them an extra blanket.

-Don't forget to lower the bed back to the lowest setting when you are done.

Tips for dealing with urine

-If your patient is on strict i/o (pronounced i and o's) you must make sure that there is a 'high hat' in the toilet. A 'high hat' it's a plastic bowl-like thing that has a wide brim (this is what makes it look like a 'hat'). The brim rest on the toilet rim under the toilet seat. It catches the urine so that it can be measured (it has graduated markings on it) and assess before it is emptied into the toilet and flushed away. You must document the amount as 'output'. In some facilities, the I/o sheet is posted on the hospital door.

-You should document and report to the nurse any of the following findings related to urine: very dark, very foamy, turbid (urine doesn't look clear), strong foul odor, appears to have blood in it, urine output of less that 30 ml/hour.

-If your patient has a foley catheter, you must empty the foley bag into a graduated container for accurate measuring. Though the bag does have graduated measurements on it, they don't always give an accurate measurement. All the same assessment finding listed above apply to the catheterize patient as well.

-The best advise I ever received when it comes to catheterizing a female is to "aim high" this way if you overshoot the urethral meatus (exterior opening of the urethra) you just adjust slightly downward. Remember, you are standing at the bedside and you have an oblique view, the urethral meatus is small and not always obviously visible. If the tip of the catheter touches above the meatus you can continue, because you cleaned this area with benadine, but if you aim too low and accidentally enter the vagina, you have contaminated the catheter and you must get a new sterile catheter.

-Catheterizing males is usually a lot easier, but occasionally, if they have BPH (Benign prostatic hyperplasia) you will meet resistance. Do not try to force the catheter to advance. Withdraw the catheter and allow a more experience handle this one. They will use a Coude-tipped catheter, it's a catheter with a curved tip that is made for patients with PBH. The nurse with experience using this type of catheter can demonstrate to you how to use this devise.

-Catheterized patients require catheter care to reduce the risks of catheter related UTI (urinary tract infection). Find out the facility's protocol for this. If your clinical patient has a catheter, ask your nurse if you can observe her doing the catheter care. This is a good chance to learn this important skill.

Tips for dealing with blood (specifically as it relates to drawing blood for labs):

-Usually the lab sheets will indicate what colored top tube you need to use for collecting blood samples. The colors of the tube top indicates whether there is a preservative in the tube, or citrate to keep the blood from clotting etc. Some lab tests require the blood to clot and separate from the plasma. Others need the blood to be Un-clotted. Phlebotomy is a fascinating practice all on it's own and many facilities have phlebotomist on staff who can do even the most difficult blood draw.

-If you patient already has a patent (open) IV, picc line, or any other type of access, ask your instructor or the nurse how to draw blood from these sites. You will have to be very careful when drawing blood from these access sites because it is very easy to introduce bacteria into the patient's circulation from these sites. That can quickly lead to potentially fatal sepsis.

-Never draw blood from the arm that is on the same side as a mastectomy. The reason is that lymph nodes are usually taken from the axilla (armpit area). This can cause this arm to have impaired circulation, a tendency to retain fluid and a possible greater risk for developing infection. There should always be a sign in the patient's room alerting staff not to use this arm for phlebotomy or taking blood pressure. If this sigh is not present, bring it to the attention of your instructor and the nurse.

-Unlike a conventional blood draw, drawing blood from these sites will require that a 'waste tube' be drawn. This tube of blood is discarded because it is very likely contaminated with IV fluid and iv meds, the next tube is the actual sample, because is it drawn off the circulating blood volume and should give accurate lab results. After, drawing the sample, you must flush the line with saline, so that the access site stays patent. Leaving blood in the line, can cause the site to clot off. Using these sites saves your patient from the pain of an additional needle sticks. These folks are already sick, preventing them any additional pain and discomfort is a good thing.

-Label the tubes with the date, time and your initials, make sure a label with the patient info is on the tube. These labels are usually on the lab order sheet. If they are not there, there should be sheets with labels in the patient's chart. Make sure that they get to the lab asap.

-Blood gas draws are done by a respiratory therapist. They are routinely done on ventilated patients and based on the results, ventilator settings can be adjusted. They are usually drawn off the radial artery. It's really cool. Don't miss the chance to see a blood gas being drawn. FYI, blood gas draws are also done in the ER in emergency situations. they give the ER doc insight into how adequate a patient's ventilation status is (ability to move o2 in and co2 out of the lungs). inadequate ventilation can quickly cause damage to the brain and can throw the blood PH so far out of whack that it can be incompatible with life. the blood gas results allow the doc to take quick action to correct them. in the ER blood glasses are usually drawn off the femoral artery.

Also I wanted to throw in a few points related to blood transfusions.
-Blood is only transfused with normal saline.
-A unit of blood must be double checked by two RNs before it is administered. As a nursing student, you can observe this process, but you cannot be one of the two nurses doing the double check.
-O negative is the universal donor: everyone can receive this type blood. In emergent situations when there is no time for typing and coss-matching, doc will request units of 'o neg'.
-AB+ is considered the universal recipient because people with this blood type can receive any type of blood.
- You must take baseline vitals before the administration.
-You must stay with your patient during the first 15 minutes of the transfusion. This is when transfusion reactions typically occur.
- A unit of blood must be transfused within 4 hrs from the time it was picked up from the blood bank, so time is of the essence when you have to give your patient blood.

You will learn a lot more about the types of reactions a patient can have during a transfusion. What are the symptoms and what are the actions you should take. It's a fascinating process and you will definitely have clinical patients who will receive blood.

when patients die

In my final senior semester I got to do three clinicals in a CCU (cardiac care unit). These were the most challenging and interesting clinicals I did during nursing school. I loved the experience. My instructor was Ms.S. She seemed to be the youngest clinical instructor I had ever had (and no, I didn't ask her age!) She was energetic, smart and funny. One of the things I was most in awe of in Ms.S, was the fact that she could move thru the CCU with such confidence and calm. I really envied that. I was eager to learn but I was also scared being on a unit with so many seriously ill patients.

Ms.S allowed us to pick our clinical assignments for ourselves. When I got the unit for my first pre-clinical, I could see that all of my other classmates had gotten there before me and chosen their assignments. I worried that I would be left with a boring uninteresting assignment. I ask a nurse working on the unit if there were any interesting patients what weren't chosen. He quickly looked at the list, and pointed to one,"He's the sickest patient in here." He nodded toward a corner room down the hall.

I went down the hall and peered into the room. The patient lay in the bed, on a ventilator and surrounded by beeping and blinking monitors and infusion pumps. His thick chart was on the small portable desk outside his room. I sat down and began to read why the patient was here.

The patient was a heavy drinker, who was found to be having a seizure. After the seizure, he was unresponsive. The patient was transported to the local hospital in a rural community.

While there ,they were trying to sort out his condition when the patient came up positive for cardiac enzymes, which meant they had had a heart attack on top of whatever else was going on. That was why the patient was transferred to the CCU where I was doing my clinicals. They had been there for about a week and this is what the doctors had learned so far about his condition. The patient had meningitis caused by psuedomonas. Psdudomonas is one scary bacterium that is resistant to almost all antibiotics and he had it running loose in his cerebral spinal fluid. The patient had cirrhosis, with high ammonia levels. This could cause encephalopathy. so the patient had two serious conditions that were directly assaulting his brain. The patent also had emphasema, heart failure, a blood clot, and the patient's kidneys where showing signs of failure. Any of these conditions alone could kill a person and this patient had them all. Slowly it was dawning on me that this patient might be too sick to get better. So many of the organ systems were under assault, and with the patient's age and the fact that they were not in the best of health before they got sick....They may not have the strength to overcome all these problems..... But I pushed those thoughts away. "I'm a nursing student not a doctor"! I scolded myself.

I gathered the data I needed to complete my pre-clinical paperwork and headed home. One thing I was sure of, I would learn a lot caring for this patient. Little did I know just how much.

I was back at the hospital early for my clinical. I was the first student to arrive. The unit was still dark, most of the patients sleeping, or what passes for sleep in the CCU.

The 7pm-7am nurse was still there. He told me that the patient had had a good night. There was no change in the patient's condition. I met the nurse who would be doing the 7am-7pm shift. She was very friendly. She seemed genuinely happy to have me working with her for the next 6 hrs. As we began to assess the patient, She began to ask me questions. She was clearly trying to see how much I knew about the nursing care the patient would require and if I understood the nature of the conditions he had. She seemed happy with my answers and in some cases surprised that I knew so much. I was glad and inwardly glowed with pride. Perhaps, I really could work in the critical care setting. My clinical day was off to a good start.

Around 9am, that patient's family arrived. They were very friendly and gracious. The nurse told them that the patient had a good night and there was no change. The family seemed to take this as good news. They stood on each side of the bed and each clasped the patient's hands. They took turns talking to him. They asked him to open his eyes and squeeze their hands. They each told him, "We need you to get better." They spent the next hour and a half talking to each other and to the patient, until finally, the doctor arrived to do rounds.

The family looked at the doctor so expectantly. It was so obvious that they were hoping for good news. The only thing the doctor said was, "We are doing everything we can. He is very sick" He spoke in a quiet, somber tone. The subtext was unmistakable, the doctor was not optimistic for the patient. One of the family bowed her head and sobbed.

I found it so awkward. Here I was, a total stranger, witnesses a profoundly painful moment in this person's life. I could only offer her kindness, a cup of water, a box of tissues. There was nothing I could do for the pain these people were feeling.

As I cared for my patient, that day, I couldn't help but think that he would probably die soon. I wondered what the journey from this existence to the next, would be like for him. Would he be relieved to be free from his ailing and sick body? Was the soul already well on it's way, even as we continued to care for the body?

The family had elected to make him a full code. This meant that if the patient stopped breathing or his heart stopped, we would do everything we could to bring him back. CPR, drugs, shocking him. Many nurses and doctors are conflicted when very sick patients are full code. No one wants to cause a very sick, dying patient's last moments full of pain and terror surrounded by well meaning strangers doing compressions and usually breaking ribs in the process, pushing drugs into their veins and shocking them. There is a fine line between helping and hurting. The worry of crossing that line is something that nurses dread.

And then there is the issue of the quality of life that the patient is being brought back to. At this point, it becomes clear that sometimes, what we are doing is really not for the benefit of the patient, but to give the family time to come to terms with the reality of their loved one's condition, and that the process of loss and grief is inevitable.

I really did learned a lot caring for my patient that day, but I was drained and eager to get away from the tragic scene in that room, when my six hours were done.

Two weeks later, as I entered the CCU for my second pre-clinical, I was surprised to see the patient's family on their way out of the unit. I managed to hide my shock as I said hello to them and then quickly walked back to the corner room. There was the patient. He looked thinner, and he was still on the ventilator, but he looked....Better. I quickly called my instructor and asked her if I could select him as my assignment for the second time. She said she would allow it this time, but for my third clinical I would have to choose a different patient.

I reviewed the patient's chart. The meningitis was resolved, his blood pressure was within an acceptable range, his kidneys were functioning within normal limits and he was to begin weaning from the ventilator. I was amazed and felt kind of ashamed. I, along with the doctor and staff had had no faith in this patient's ability to overcome his conditions. We were all wrong to not have had more faith in him and in ourselves, because his recovery was also a testament to the excellent, and diligent care he had received.

The next day, I was leaning over the bed, listening to my patients heart and lung sounds, I glanced up. He was looking me straight in the eye. His eyes were focused. It was clear that he was alert and oriented. I grasped his hand, and told him who I was and that I had help to take care of him when he was really sick. I told him that I was so glad that he was doing better. He squeezed my hand in reply.

On my third and final pre-clincal in the CCU, the first thing I did was peek into the patient's room. The patient was sleeping peacefully. The ventilator was gone, there was only one bag of IV fluid infusing at a slow rate. The nurse told me the patient was due to transfer out to a rehab facility. I was still so amazed at his recovery.

I walked down the hall toward the dry erase board where all the patient's on the unit were listed. There was a newly admitted patient. I went to the door of the patient's room and ask the nurse as he come out.
"Would be okay for me to choose her for my clinical assignment?"
He shrugged.
"Sure, she has some issue with her heart, but we don't know exactly what is going on. She went to her doctor due to weakness and chest pain. He had her transported here. She's negative for cardiac enzymes. I'm preparing her to go down to CAT scan."

I went into the patient's room. The patient was very pale and appeared to be very sick. I introduced myself and told her that I wanted to help take care of her the next day, if that was okay with her. She weakly nodded and curled a frail hand on her chest and whispered "hurts."

I left the room and told the nurse she was complaining of chest pain. I followed as he went into the room. As he began to talk to the patient, the patient pulled out her IV. The patient's eyes vacantly scanned across the room not focusing on anything, the patient's thin arm dripped blood across the linen. The nurse quickly tore open some 4x4s and applied pressure to the bleeding IV site. Another

nurse came in and took over holding the gauze in place. While the patient's nurse quickly started a new IV in the other arm, then he placed a portable monitor on the gurney next to the patient. By then, another nurse was waiting transport the patient to CAT scan. The nurse informed her that that the patient had just become confused and pulled out their IV, he continues to give report as they pushed the gurney thru the double doors of the unit. The doors swung closed with a "swoosh". They were gone.

I sat down and started going thru the patient's chart. It was very thin. I was glad that the patient was in the hospital. The patient was clearly very sick and something was very wrong. Negative troponin, so she didn't have a heart attack. But she had a family history of heart disease, and the patient was post menopausal, so she was at risk for a heart attack. Women sometimes present differently than the classic heart attack
symptoms, but the negative troponin meant that none ofthe cardiac muscle cells were damaged. It was a puzzle. Oh well, I thought to myself, at least the patient is being monitored and the CAT scan will probably give the doctors a good idea what is going on. I was confident that by morning, the doctors would have instituted a plan of action to treat whatever was ailing the patient. I gathered my notes and left.

As I walked into the unit the next morning, I immediately saw that my patient's room was empty. The bed was neatly made and set on the highest level, ready for a new patient to be transferred onto it from a transport gurney. I went over to the dry erase board. The patient's name was not on it. Damn! They must have been transferred out. Now I will have to select a new patient.

I approached a nurse sitting behind the nurses station.
"Do you know what happened with my patient in bed 1?"
He looked up from his charting.
"Hum.....Oh yeah, she died."
He went back to his charting.
I waited a few seconds for him to chuckle and say he was just joking. You see, teasing nursing students is a sport for most experienced nurses, but he just continued to chart.

I realized that he was serious. My patient had really died! How could that be? Yes, she was sick, but she was nowhere near as sick as the other patient and he recovered. I can't believe it!

I walked out of the unit, took out my cell phone and called my instructor to tell her something that I never really believed I would have to say during nursing school, "My patient died".

When my instructor came in, she started asking around the unit and eventually she put together what happened with my patient. I was trying to go thru my newly assigned patient's chart, when she came to tell me what happened.

The CAT scan revealed that my patient had an aortic dissection. The aortic is the great vessel that is first to receive oxygenated blood that is pumped by the left ventricle out into the systemic circulation. Of all the vessels in the body, it receives the greatest pressure because it receives blood pumped at full force from the heart. If there is a weakened spot in the aorta, it tends to become weaker and weaker. Remember the heart is pumping constantly, so a weakened area in the aorta gets no chance to repair itself. Instead, the continuous pumping pressure erodes the weakened spot more and more, and if not caught soon enough and surgically repaired, it will rupture.

My patient was immediately taken from CAT scan to surgery, but as soon as their chest was opened, the aorta ruptured and the patient died.

I realized that the episode of confusion that they had on their way down to CAT scan was probably a manifestation of the dissection worsening. I realized that they had probably died before I even got home the day before and I realized that my fretting over the other patient dying was a waste of time, and that short of having x-ray (or CAT scan) vision, there was no way I could have known how imminent my patient's death was. So, yes, from time to time I probably will fret and worry over patients that are seriously ill, but I realized that I really serve my patients best by always trying to focus on my job as a nurse and doing everything I can for them. That is something I have control over, because even with all our amazing technology and our vast body of medical knowledge, sometimes who lives and who dies can be out of our hands.

Choosing a specialty

Another great thing about clinicals is that they can help you chose a specialty. There are so many different types of nursing out there that deal with so many different aspects of health care, there is something that that will be just the right fit for you. The only thing you have to do is keep an open mind and be willing to explore the possibilities.

Now as for the whole 'open mind' thing, well, I have to make a confession. There are some specialties of nursing that I absolutely do not want to go into. There are three and I'll explain why.

The first is psychiatric nursing. The reason is that I have enough crazy people in my family that I have to deal with, that I have zero desire to deal with more. I know that sounds mean, but the thought of trying to heal emotional, and psychological wounds leaves me feeling helpless and overwhelmed. It's not something I'm proud of but it is the truth. I'd much rather deal with the wounds and illness of the body. I have more confidence in applying my nursing knowledge in that area.

I did have some nursing instructors who specialized in this field and they all said the same thing, they were very surprised to find that they loved psych nursing. So, who knows, perhaps one day I may find my self having a change of heart when it comes to psych nursing, but for now....No thank-you.

The next, is working in a burn unit.

Nursing textbooks have no shortage of gruesome photographs, but the one's that always got to me were the ones in the burn chapter. I guess because lot of them were of children. The nurses in the burn unit deal with very sick people/kids who are in a lot of pain, and who are facing a long uphill road to recovery. If they recovery, many of them face dealing with permanent disfigurement. In other words, it's a sad situation in the beginning and can be a sad situation in the end.

A very important part of the treatment of burns is a process known as 'debridement'. This is the process of removing dead tissue, and purulent slough usually caused by psuedomonas bacteria. This bug has a real affinity for burn wounds, it causes a green foul smelling slime to form. It must be scrubbed off. As you can imagine this is agonizingly painful for the patient as well as the nurse. It takes a special kind of fortitude to work in a burn unit. Honestly, I'm not sure I could do it.

The next is working in a NICU. This one is my own particular pet peeve: nursing students who go all gaga-eyed when they say they want to work in a nicu. It's like they think it will be like being in a diaper commercial except they will be wearing scrubs and the babies will be really small and in incubators. They clearly think it's going to be so much fun.

What bothers me is that these students are really not thinking about the job realistically.

Every job, no matter what, will have bad days. I really don't think these nursing students are considering what constitutes a bad day when you work in the NICU. It's this: a baby dies and you get to watch parents go thru the most devastating loss that there is. That doesn't sound like fun to me.

Then there are the other bad days, when you watch over a baby that has been abandoned or a baby that is dying from a skull fracture, because the mom was holding the baby and smoking crack. She dropped the baby but not the crack pipe; or you are about to discharge a baby to the care of her 15 year old mother, who never got any prenatal care and who you seriously doubt has a clue how to care for baby. Try to go home and get a good night sleep after any of those days.

And the babies are not just the only patients, you have to deal with the parents too. Parents who are literally worried sick. Moms who are dealing with all the hormonal upheaval that comes with giving birth and now with the fact that there is a complication that has landed their baby in the NICU. Hysterical, weeping, totally freaked out parents. You have to deal with them too. And you thought you avoided psyche nursing!

Please, take my advise, when you are seriously considering a specialty, find a nurse that is working in that specialty and ask them, "What is a bad day like in the NICU...., the ICU...., the burn unit... etc.

Anyone can handle the good days, the average days. It's the bad days, that really test you as a nurse and a person. If you are not prepared and equipped to handle the bad days in your specialty, you will be on a downward spiral to burn out. It's better to find out what it's like first.

Doing nursing school when you are a single parent

When I had finally gotten my nursing school application in the mail, I heard through the grape vine that one of the instructors conducting orientation for the new in coming class, told those brand new eager nursing student, that they needed to say "good-bye" to their husbands, wives and children for the next year and a half. They were going to be too busy to function in those capacities while in nursing school.

When I heard this I was appalled and really mad. Does being a parent mean you should not peruse a career in nursing??? Well, I'm a single mom and I managed to complete nursing school and get my degree and I did it while being an attentive and caring mom to my three kids. So don't let anyone tell you that you can't do nursing school and be a single parent.

Was it hard? You betcha! Looking back on it sometimes I don"t know how I did it, but I can tell you a few things that can help.

First of all, being a parent can actually give you an edge because nursing school and parenting are a lot alike:

-Both require you to do things you HAVE TO DO whether you want to or not.
-Both require maturity and discipline.
-Both require that you care for people who can't care for themselves.

-Both are kind of like clubs in that only another parent can understand what its like to be a parent, and only a nursing student can understand what life is like for a nursing student.
-Both are transformative experiences.
-Both consist of doing a huge number of tasks (many unpleasant) for the well being of others.

One of the biggest challenges the nursing student/parent will face is: CHILDCARE!

Unless you are married and your spouse's schedule allows them to take over child care when your crazy clinical schedule takes over your life, get use to the fact that you will have multiple baby-sitters during the time you are in nursing school.

Hire a sitter, unless you have friends and or family who are BEGGING to watch your kids. Asking friends and family to watch your kids can cause a lot of tension and resentment. This will just create MORE STRESS for you to deal with and that is the last thing that you will need. While other folks may love your kids, they may not want to take on the responsibility of watching your kids hours at a time. Hiring a sitter means that you both can have a clear understanding of what you can both expect from each other.

Have a list of MUSTS: MUST speak some english. MUST have reliable transportation. MUST not be allergic to your household pets. Must be a non-smoker (or at the very least, understand that they cannot smoke in your house. You may also need to make it clear that they should not leave cigarette butts in your driveway, flower beds, front lawn etc. I once left a collection of cigarette butts on my kitchen counter so one of my sitters would get a clue about how to properly dispose of her cigarette butts) MUST understand that certain rooms of your house are of limits. I once admired my babysitter's toe nails that were painted a vivid pink. She told me that she had BORROWED MY NAIL POLISH! This meant that she had been in my master bath going thru my draws to find where I kept my nail polish-ugh!! A list of MUSTs can nip a lot of inappropriateness in the bud.

If you want your sitter to do light housekeeping, you will need to be specific about what you consider light housekeeping. You may consider that to be washing dishes and picking up the floor, but your sitter might think that means that the house is just shy of a total garbage dump.

Pay your sitter at the end of the work week. Occasionally your babysitter will have a situation come up and will ask to be paid early. It can work to your benefit to be flexible and do this once in a while, but otherwise pay them only at the end of the week.

When I was in nursing school, I had a lot of sitters. Some left because they got new jobs. Unfortunately, some of the best sitters you will have are folks who are waiting for a better opportunity to come along. It's sad when they leave, but you can't help but be happy that they have the opportunity to do what they really want to be doing.

Then there are other more unpleasant reasons that a sitter leaves your employ. I had one sitter who quickly figured out that she was an essential part of my pursuit of a nursing degree. She thought she could use that as leverage to demand more money. She clearly thought she had me over a barrel and she would have, except for the fact that when I advertise for a sitter, I keep a folder of all the applicant e-mails for the job. I quickly fired off a few e-mails and soon had a short list of folks who were still interested in the job. I set up a few quick interviews and hired a new sitter. So I had a new sitter who wanted the job as badly as I needed someone to do the job and was willing to accept the pay that I could afford to pay.

Since I was not working, the only money I had was what was left over from my financial aid. This money had to cover our household bills and pay the sitter. I paid my sitters really well to compensate for the crazy schedule that nursing students have to adhere to. For a Monday morning, when I needed the sitter to be at my house at 6 am, so I could get to my 7 am clinical on time. The sitter would have to get the kids dressed, fed and on the school bus. This would mean, that in the fall and winter, the sitter would actually only have to work a few hours in the early morning when I had to get to a clinical. For a morning, I'd set a lump sum amount. this compensated the sitter for getting out of bed early and working the 2 hours I needed. Paying hourly makes more sense when you need a lot of hours from your sitter. This is true during the summer when your kids are out of school or if your kids are not yet in school.

You should also try work out an arrangement for your sitter to pick up your child from school if they get sick. (For this, remember to put your sitter on the official pick-up list at the school.)

I was always on high alert for my kids getting sick. At the first sign of sore throat, cough, sniffles or fever, I would get everyone in the car and to the doctor to be examined and especially swabbed for Strep. I would try to get everyone to the doc by Thursday, Friday the very latest. This would mean that if they were put on antibiotics, they would have the weekend for the antibiotics to kick in. This would also mean that come Monday, even if they were not 100%, I could write a note explaining that they had been to the doctor are were: a) on antibiotics or b) negative for strep or c) just suffering from a regular cold virus that would just have to run it's course.

Unfortunately, the school will only let your kid return to school if they know you have taken the kid to the doctor, and if you take your kid to the doctor, your kid will probably end up on antibiotics.

During the years I was in nursing school, my kids ended up on antibiotics much more than I would have liked but telling a teacher that my kids was on antibiotic were magic words that would allow my kid to return to school, and allow me to complete a clinical that cannot be rescheduled. If I were to miss the clinical, I would fail the semester, regardless of how perfect a grade I had in my theory classes.

It was an unfair, unpleasant fact of life I had to live with while I was in nursing school. The irony was that the kid actually got the bug from the school, but the school views a sick kid as a petri dish of infection. As if the child brewed up the infection all on their own! I even once had an elementary school teacher tell me that she tries to stay away anyone who might be sick! Didn't she realize that that could be each and every kid in her school? Didn't she consider that when she was making her career choice? Yikes!

Perhaps nursing isn't for me after all......

Once, I was doing a clinical at a hospital where I had done great clinicals on many other occasions. I had no reason to think that this particular day would be any different. I had finished up everything that I needed to do with my assigned patient, and for some reason that I can't recall now, I went into the room of a patient that was assigned to my fellow class mate A.

Upon entering the room, I immediately regretted whatever I had agreed to help A with.

The patient, a very elder woman, was sitting on the bed-side commode. The room smelled absolutely awful.

It was so bad that I was really struggling to keep my composure and was afraid that I might be ill. I tried to breath shallowly thru my mouth, but this didn't really help.

The smell was getting to me so bad and I was struggling not to loose it. My heart was pounding and I was starting to feel dizzy. I felt like I was on the verge of a full fledged panic attack. Though breathing thru my mouth aleved the smell, I felt even more revolted at the thought of inhaling that fetid miasma into my body.

I had finally, way too late, encountered the one thing that totally turned me off to nursing.

I looked at A. She was calm and completely unbothered by the smell. She chatted with me about her patient as we changed the linen on the bed. She explained that her patient was complaining of excess gas.

IT WAS JUST GAS!! I couldn't believe that GAS was getting to me. I was just one semester away from graduating and here I was, completely overwhelmed by GAS! I had seen horrific purulent wounds, witnesses multiple surgeries, cleaned rivers of urine and feces, but now GAS from a tiny elderly lady had me so overwhelmed that it was all I could do to keep myself from bolting out of the room.

Not only were my senses in an upheaval, but I was devastated as well. Clearly I was wrong, when I thought I could handle being a nurse. I had just spent over 3 years pursuing a nursing degree and now THIS! How could I ever hope to be a capable, competent nurse if I couldn't handle intestinal gas??!

I had a fake smile plastered on my pale, sweaty face, nodding as A continued to chat. I was trying my best not to let on that my dream of being a nurse, was at that moment, spiraling down the drain.

There was a quick knock on the door. The door opened. It was our clinical Instructor, a mature, seasoned floor nurse who had decades of nursing experience under her belt. She had seen it all twice and there was nothing that ever ruffled her professional calm demeanor.

She took one step into the room with a beaming smile on her face…but then….

A split second later, her smile morphed into a look of complete and utter revulsion and disgust. She quickly backed out of the room firmly closing the door behind her.

Now I had to try not to laugh and weep with relief. I realize that it wasn't just me!! If it got my clinical instructor it had to be bad! It wasn't just me being wimpy.

I have since learned that every nurse has something that gets to her/him. Some are fine with urine or feces, but sputum sends them into dry heaves. Some nurses are only bothered by patients with body odor. It's a very individual thing and nothing to worry about or be ashamed of. (Oddly enough, nurses love to talk about what grosses them out!)

So don't let the fact that there is something in nursing that you find hard to stomach, deter you from pursuing a career in nursing. All nurses get grossed out from time to time. We are just very good at not letting it show.

Your preceptor and you: not always a match made in heaven.

Your last semester in school will be largely devoted to your preceptorship. You will be assigned a preceptor at the facility you choose to do your preceptorship at. You may be asked to list two choices, so if your first choice doesn't work out you will have a second place you can do your preceptorship.

It is wise to do your preceptorship at a facility that you would like to work in. It is even wiser to do your preceptorship in a facility that is known for hiring new grads (the job offer is contingent upon you passing the state board exam and getting your license). Just because you have a brand RN license, doesn't mean that every hospital and facility will be lining up to hire you. The nursing shortage is a shortage of EXPERIENCED nurses. Hiring new grads can be expensive and risky for hospitals.

You need to start thinking about where you want to do your preceptorship at least the semester before you will have to do your preceptorship and you should definitely look at your preceptorship as a stepping stone to getting your first job.

Landing that first job and getting that first year of experience under your belt can be daunting and many new grads struggle to find jobs. For this reason, it may be worth it to choose a preceptorship site that involves a little driving, if it means you stand a good shot at being offered a job.

You will have to do a little investigating to find out the best place to do your preceptorship. A good way to go about it is to ask members of the graduating class, if anyone got job offers when doing their preceptorship (nursing students will be so excited by a job offer that it is IMPOSSIBLE for then to NOT share this news with their fellow classmates). I

t's common for hospitals that are new grad-friendly to offer jobs to students that precept with them. This makes sense because they get to train you but don't have to pay you during this process and observe how well you function as a novice nurse.

You can also ask the instructor who teaches the final semester what hospitals offered jobs to students.

Why all the hustle to try to get that first job? When you get your first job, for the first year, you are labeled a NOVICE NURSE. This is a good thing in that you will hopefully not be thrown into the deep end and put into nursings situation that you are not ready for. Most experienced nurses will take you under their wing and be happy to teach you things that took them years to learn and they are always a sounding board for you to bounce ideas off of whenever you are not sure about your new fledgling nursing judgement.

The bad thing is that your opportunities are limited until you get that first year of experience. Once you have a year of experience, you can transfer to a different unit, do travel nursing, look for a job at a hospital closer to home ect.

The absolute worst thing about being a novice nurse is that you are an easy target for MEAN NURSES. They will mock you and sneer at your questions. They will enjoy rapid firing questions at you just to get you flustered and trip you up. You have to stick up for yourself and not get upset or defensive. Mean Nurses are a tiny minority of nurses, most of the nurses you will meet and work with are wonderful people. (Also just FYI, mean nurses never last, they never stick around for long. After a while they are so isolated, alone and miserable that they leave for new jobs.)

Now a cautionary tale: This did not happen to me, but it did happen to another nursing student. It's the kind of situation that can keep poor-about-to-graduate nursing student awake at night with the lights on.

Usually, you DO get to pick where you do your preceptorship, you DO NOT get to pick your preceptor.

Now just imagine, that you meet your preceptor and you dislike each other on site. Everything one of you says, rubs the other the wrong way. Your personalities clash in a way that would mean that you two would never willingly choose to be in the same room together. Now imagine that there are no other places for you to do your preceptor ship.

What do you do?

You could try to hustle and find yourself another preceptorship site with a new preceptor, but it's unlikely when you consider that you have to allow yourself time to start and complete your preceptorship hours and the days and times you have free to do them may be limited if you are working, or are a parent with children you have to care for too (a single parent has this compounded because they don't have a spouse to pass this responsibility off to occasionally) and you can only do your preceptorship on the days your preceptor works.

You can postpone graduating which means you will have to take an F for the semester. (Not liking your preceptor is not a special circumstance that would incline the administration to let you leave the program for a semester with no penalty.) Not completing your preceptorship would mean you would fail clinicals and you would not be able to progress with the program. You would have to apply for remediation a non-credit review type course. A spot in the remediation class could not be guaranteed, but upon completion of the remediation you could reapply for the program and possibly be readmitted, if your GPA was still high enough to qualify for the program. You will end up graduating 2 semesters behind your classmates.

This is what happened to a friend, but there is another option.

you can suck it up and do whatever it takes to get along with your preceptor.

You will not complain about your preceptor to the other nurses on the unit, but instead have nothing but praise for your preceptor. Thank your preceptor for every skill she teaches you and every time she corrects you. You will do every task with a good attitude and do your very best to win over your preceptor. You will remind yourself constantly that your preceptor's evaluation can either pass you or fail you.

This will be your first lesson learning how to get along with incredibly difficult and unpleasant people. Because that is invaluable skill in nursing and one you will put to good use many many times in your nursing career, trust me. (Unless your patient is in the hospital to have a baby, chances are, they are not happy or excited to be there, so you are dealing with people who would rather be anywhere else than in a hospital talking to you.)

With some planning and effort you can make the last and most challenging semester of nursing school a success.

taking the NCLEX

There two things that I was the 'first' at in nursing school. I was the first to ace a calculations test.

In all honesty it was only 3 questions, but it was given during my classes' orientation for incoming new students. Not only did I get all questions right, I was the only person to get them right out of 52 students.

The reason was I had completed the whole dosage calculations textbook before I even took my first nursing class. (I still had plenty of things to stress over in nursing school, but the calculations tests were not one).

The second was that I was the first to get my RN license. The day after I had taken my final, final exam in nursing school, I knew that I finally qualified to take the NYCLEX. I wanted to register as soon as possible because I thought I might have to wait months before I would finally be scheduled to take it. Most of my class had no plans to take the exam anytime soon, but instead were enrolling in nclex prep courses. The last thing I wanted was to be back in a class room. I decided that I would study and prepare the best I could on my own.

After registering to take the test, a calendar pop-up window opened. It showed all the days that the exam was being given. I could choose which day to take the exam. I choses to take it the following week. There was a part of me that thought I was totally crazy to take the exam so soon, but I also knew that the info I learned in nursing school would never be fresher in my mind than it was at that time.

Once I got to the testing site I began to think that I had made a huge mistake. I heard many of the other folks there to take the test comment that, 'they were sure they would pass this time.'....Yikes!

I learned quickly not to keep my hand on the mouse. Once you clicked an answer, it went to the next and there was no going back.

The questions were bare bones, with very little in the way of back story in the scenarios. Many times, more than one answer seemed like it could be right. I had to really pick the answers apart to eliminate them and what was left had to be the right answer, though I never felt 100% sure.

I plodded thru questions like this for over an hour and then suddenly then computer shut off. Unlike taking an exam in nursing school, I had no idea how I had done. I was left with the sinking problem that I had done really poorly, probably failed even.

I was so upset that I did the only thing that I knew would give me some peace of mind. I did THE TRICK.

When you register to take the NYCLEX you have to pay to take the exam. If you failed you will have to retake the exam and that means you will have to pay another fee. So if you go to reregister to take the exam and you are prompted to pay the exam fee, you will know that you failed and must retake the test. If you are not allowed pay for a retest, this means that you passed. I was not allowed to pay. So I knew that despite my worry, I had passed the NYCLEX and I was finally a licensed registered nurse.

Just remember that everyone leaves the NYCLEX upset and worried. It doesn't mean that you failed.

That's all for now....

I truly hope that I've given you some tips and insights that will be helpful as you begin or consider beginning a nursing program. Good luck and best wishes!!

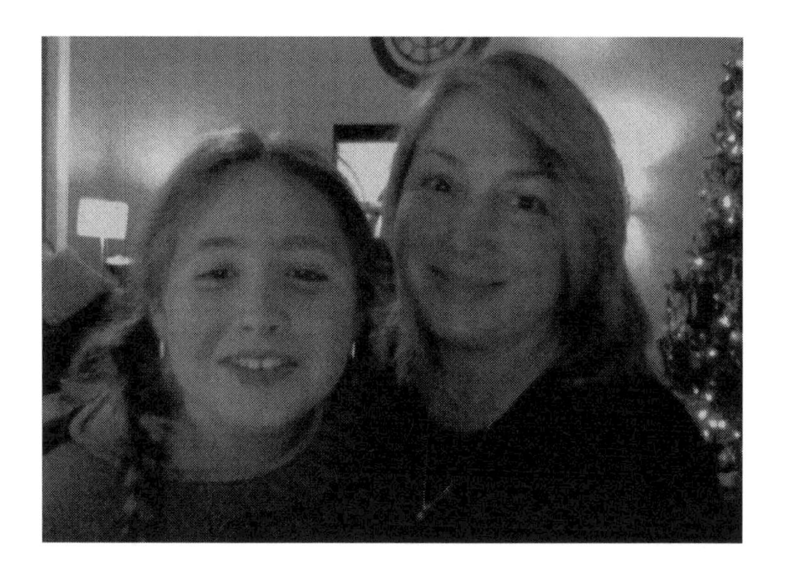

Stacey Bernikow lives in Alabama and is the lucky mom of three awesome kids, Leah, Jake and Rose. She also lives with Kinkaju and Skippy, the family cat and dog. They are pretty awesome too. She currently works on a busy Med/Surg unit. She loves her job.

Made in the USA
Middletown, DE
14 November 2016